TERRY FOX

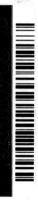

Terry Fox

A Pictorial Tribute
To The Marathon
Of Hope

by Jeremy Brown and Gail Harvey

Published by
General Publishing Co. Limited
Don Mills, Ontario

Distributed by
PaperJacks Ltd.
Markham, Ontario

Copyright © 1980
The Brownstone Press Limited
Toronto, Ontario

This book is a tribute to the heroic achievement of Terry Fox. The sum of fifty cents per copy sold or the audited profit, whichever is greater, will be donated by General Publishing Co. Limited to research in the fight against cancer.

First published in 1980 by
General Publishing Co. Limited
Don Mills, Ontario

and distributed by
PaperJacks Limited
330 Steelcase Road East
Markham, Ontario

First Printing, 100,000 copies
Second Printing, 50,000 copies

Canadian Cataloguing in Publication Data
Brown, Jeremy, 1932
Terry Fox
ISBN 0-7701-0176-3 (pbk.)
I. Fox, Terry, 1958- II. Cancer-Biography.
III Runners (Sports)-Canada-Biography.
I. Harvey, Gail. II. Title.

RC263.B76   616.99'471'0924   C81-094110-4

Printed and Bound in Canada
0-7701-0176-3

To Terry Fox

For what he has given to Canada and to the world.

ACKNOWLEDGMENTS

My collaborator on this book is Gail Harvey, a staff photographer for United Press Canada. Her first sight of Terry Fox running down University Avenue in Toronto triggered the feeling of "wonder and disbelief" that resulted in her using her spare time to document the run. Her skill and compassion are evident in the photographs throughout this pictorial record. Many other excellent photographers contributed, but it is Gail's efforts photographically, and her diligence as a photo editor, that made the book possible.

To produce a work such as this in the short time allowed required enormous dedication. Fay Matthews worked tirelessly rooting out photographs, air expressed in from both ends of the country, and unearthing material about our extraordinary subject. Susan Barrable supervised the production and kept the enterprise on schedule. The brilliant artist and caricaturist, Andy Donato of the *Toronto Sun*, designed the pages, while Vince Desai executed the layouts and fine-tuned the displays.

There must be special mention of one person whose lively wit and great humanity helped not only the Marathon of Hope, but this project as well. He is Bill Vigars who was seconded from the Ontario division of the Canadian Cancer Society. He had accompanied Terry from Montreal to that sad and momentous day in Thunder Bay. Over the years as a professional journalist I have met scores of 'advance men', publicists and tour managers. In those roles Bill Vigars stands supreme. He orchestrated not only the details as the run unfolded, but also the larger impact that developed. He formed a close relationship with Terry, and his understanding and love helped us all. He is a very special person.

My thanks also to Bill Ballentine, vice-president and station manager of radio station CKFM, and Jerry Good, vice-president of programming. They provided the time for this project, as well as the encouragement, facilities and understanding that resulted in close to $500,000 being donated through the station to the Terry Fox Fund. As of this writing, the total pledged and given to that fund exceeds $16,000,000.

Toronto   September 5, 1980

Hello, my name is Vivian.

I'm sending five dollers

to Terry Fox for the

cancer sosiety. I wish

him the best and all my

family (does) does. The

money came from my alowen

-ce and the money from

my brother's toothfairy.

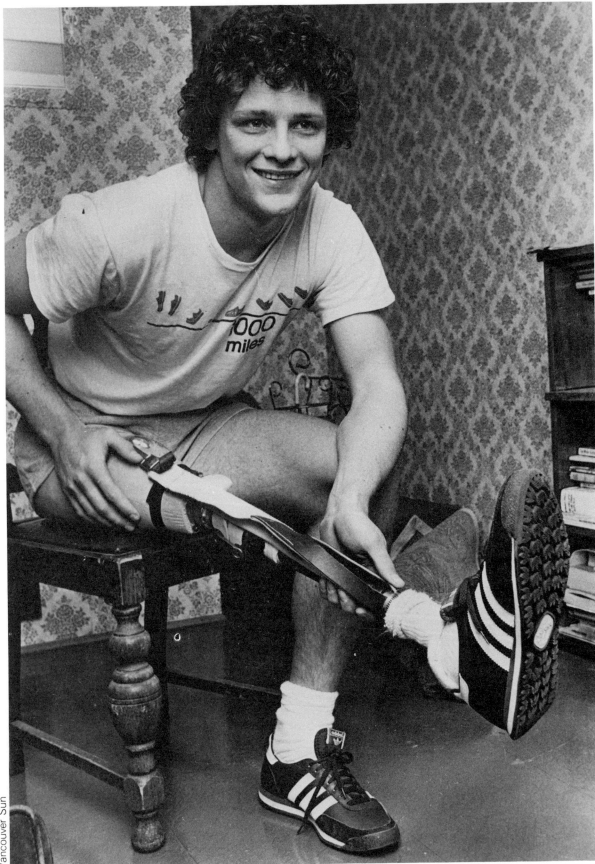

INTRODUCTION

On October 15, 1979, Terry Fox wrote the Canadian Cancer Society an eloquent and moving letter, proposing a run across Canada to raise money for research into cancer. As I reread it to prepare this introduction, I reflected on his haunting phrase, "Somewhere the hurting must stop . . . " It was an evocation of man's deepest cry, a reach into the heart and offer of help to the victims of a particularly painful and savage disease.

I reflected on that phrase again when I listened to the tape of Terry's interview, an interview from a stretcher in Thunder Bay shortly after the diagnosis that cancer had struck again, this time in both lungs. Terry, his voice cracking with emotion, simply said, "I've got to go home."

On September 2nd, a day I shall never forget, Terry's Marathon of Hope was stilled. The nation cried with him, for he had touched many hearts in a fashion few others have ever achieved. A friend in the radio station where I work broke the news quietly, in advance of the confirming call from Thunder Bay. But the advance warning of impending bad news could not cushion the terrible shock. Speechless, I railed at the hopeless injustice of it all, the unfairness of the disease randomly striking twice at this mere youth, clean of limb, clear of mind, indomitable of purpose.

Well before that awful date I had succumbed completely to the gallantry of the marathon. It had started when the manager of my station, Bill Ballentine, suggested I might look into this Marathon of Hope. I had missed the initial reports of Terry dipping his artificial leg into the Atlantic on April 12, and his progress through the Maritimes. Now he was in Quebec, and I riffled through the skimpy material available to me. I came across one photograph taken by Colin Price from the *Province,* the classic photo which captured the intensity of this handsome, tragically crippled youth. That one picture was enough to reach through the layers of cynicism, and into the soul. Things weren't quite the same after that.

After several initial broadcasts, I was invited by the Canadian Cancer Society to fly to Ottawa and meet Terry as he ran into the capital.

At 4:30 the next morning we drove out to the van which was their mobile home. There was Darrell, the younger brother who provided the counterpoint to the arduousness of the run, and Doug Alward, the driver, manager and companion. The van would be moved precisely one mile at a time, a reachable target for Terry. The sun was barely rising as Terry came over the hill, great trailer trucks virtually brushing him in their after-wind. With his strange, awkward gait, this tiny figure struck the chord I knew he would. At that moment, I cried.

My particular response was not uncommon, but others reacted in vastly different ways. My wife, not in the least tearful, saw Terry's achievement as a positive exultation, a surmounting of adversity in the most positive fashion. No tears there, no lumps in the throat, just admiration for a rare quality of determination. Terry himself did not deal in pity. He sought no pity, no compassion. I watched him, I watched as he ran, I saw him at rallies, at dinners, joking with his family and colleagues.

Perhaps his words are far better than mine. In an interview on radio station CKFM in Toronto, Judy Webb asked him the following question:

"You have moved greatly, indeed, moved to tears a lot of people in this town who are cynical, jaded and sophisticated, and in some cases pretty hard

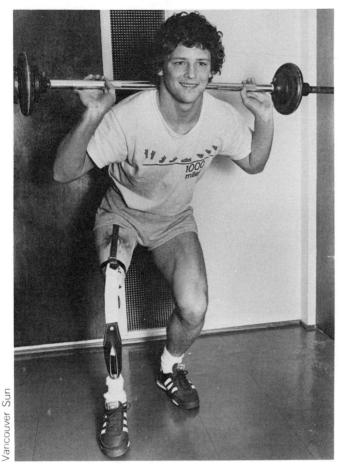

bitten. Are you concerned at all that people not feel pity for you?"

Terry responded: "If anybody feels pity for me they don't know, they don't understand what I'm doing. Yeah, that would bother me if any of those people are crying for reasons of pity. Then I'm not getting the message across and people don't understand what I'm doing because there is nobody who's happier than I am, doing what I'm doing.

"For fulfillment, the rewards that I'm getting out of doing what I'm doing are something that I don't think about. Why should somebody have any pity for me? This is the way I feel. A lot of people might feel pity because I've got one leg or because of the way I run, but it's true when I say you could take my real leg away and I'd probably be even stronger than I am now with one."

Webb: "Can you explain that?"

Terry: "To me you have to be stronger. I know that, especially since I've been through what I went through with cancer. Life now is more rewarding and challenging because I'm doing it on one leg. I don't know—just walking, playing golf, running—there is just *something* when you do it. You feel more satisfied. I feel more satisfied than I did before. I try harder than I did before.

"If you took my other leg away I would have to try harder to do things I can do on one leg, and even harder to do things with two legs the way normal people do, and when you are doing your best and becoming normal, and you're getting close to normal, you really feel happy with yourself."

This is close to the core of Terry Fox. He really *believes* every word of that statement. He is *not* crippled. No one need cry for him. No one need pity him. No one need waste a shard of emotion on his physical condition.

Why then, the outpouring of emotion? Why the incredible response, a response which cuts through the routine of the day? Why have people called me in tears after they've seen Terry run?

In the course of helping to raise money for Terry's objective, I have received hundreds of letters and phone calls. Many have come from people crippled with various diseases. He has given them inspiration and hope. There have been calls from children. His example has given them direction. Communications have come from corporate leaders, secretaries, salesmen, housewives, teachers, clerks, entrepreneurs, hustlers, from game wardens and farmers, athletes and paraplegics, cancer victims and hardy outdoorsmen, from police and restaurateurs, from every facet of our society. There is a common thread—pity notwithstanding—a common thread that Terry Fox has for a brief moment elevated all of us. The words sound simple, yet these words are all I have. His is a naive purity which flashed like a beacon across the country, a beacon which will remain permanent. Between April 12 and September 2, 1980, a legend formed, circled, and coalesced into substance. Let me say simply that Terry Fox has caught the essential spirit of what man can be.

And somewhere the hurting must stop.

Jeremy Brown
November 1980
Toronto

THE MARATHON OF HOPE BEGINS

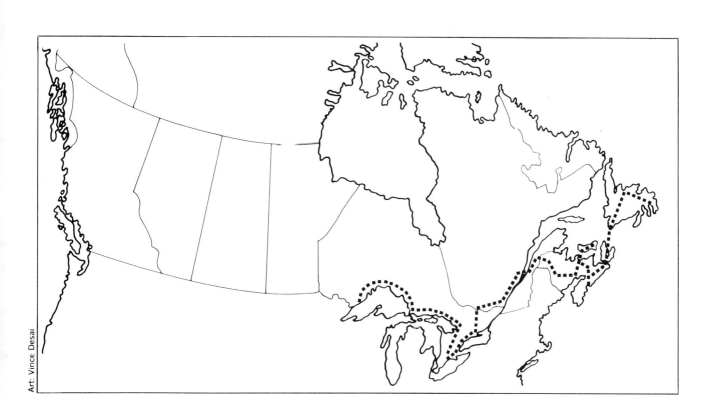

Art: Vince Desai

One morning in March of 1977, Terrence Stanley Fox, eighteen, could not get out of his bed because of a searing pain in his right knee. The night before at his high school Terry Fox had circled the track despite this same pain, a pain that had started weeks and weeks before, and would not go away.

He thought at the time it was a cartilage problem, but he didn't want to quit during the basketball season; he was a guard on the freshman basketball team at Simon Fraser University in Burnaby, British Columbia, a position he had earned through hard work and skill. On that morning in March, in the small, ranch-style home in Port Coquitlam, the pain was too great to move. His father, Rolly Fox, took him for a thorough medical examination. After a series of tests, a doctor walked into Terry's hospital room, and, with his parents standing by, Terry was told he had osteogenic sarcoma of the right knee, the most common form of a rare bone cancer. The leg must be amputated, and as soon as possible, because the cancer was dangerous and would spread quickly.

At the age of eighteen, the tragedy was enormous.

This was the Terry Fox who at first couldn't make the grade eight basketball team, but who had practised so long and so hard that he was named athlete of the year when he graduated from 'Poco'—Port Coquitlam High.

This was the Terry Fox who had applied himself with equal diligence to his studies, achieved straight *A* grades, and gained admission to university where his field of interest was kinesiology, the study of motion.

His leg? Amputated? This was far more terrifying than the thought of cancer, about which he knew little. That night, in the privacy of his room, he cried and cried. It would be the first, and last time he cried for himself. The next day his room was crowded with relatives, friends, and well-wishers.

The night before the operation, three days after the diagnosis, his former basketball coach came to see him with an article about a one-legged runner who had finished the New York Marathon. (This was the same coach who had told him years before he was too small for basketball, and should take up wrestling. "I had to eat my words," he said.)

"I had a dream that night," Terry was to say many times throughout the marathon, "that I would run right across Canada. I didn't even know if I'd be able to walk, but it was something that never left me, that dream, that fantasy."

Terry was up six weeks after the operation and soon began playing eighteen holes of golf. He also went through sixteen months of chemotherapy, therapy he began to dread. It was not the pain of the treatments that caused the dread—that was bad enough—it was the fear that at any one of the monthly examinations the doctors might discover the virulent cancer had not been eradicated through the amputation and had cropped up again. After sixteen months, there was no evidence of new cancerous growth.

During his hospital convalescence he saw much tragedy and pain in the cancer wards of the Royal Columbian Hospital in New Westminster, B.C.

In his letter to the Cancer Society about his proposed run, he wrote, "Somewhere the hurting must stop . . . " The reference was to the pain of others, the children who did not appear again after operations, the youths emaciated from cancer and pain.

In no time at all, his dream, his fantasy began to

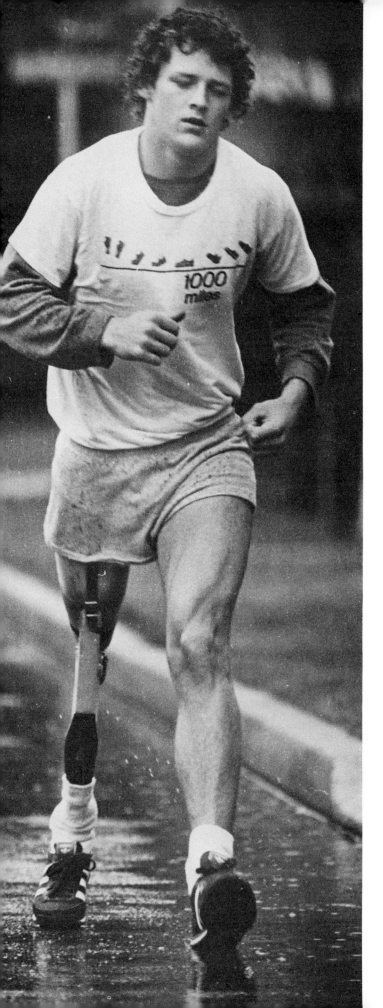

take shape. The discipline was already there. It stemmed from the competition he knew in his formative years, from the love and guidance of his parents. (As one observer said, "If there was an award for Parents of the Decade, it would go to Betty and Rolly Fox.")

In February of 1979, about two years after the operation, he began training for a run across Canada. His first run was a half of a mile. By the end of eight months he was up 13½ miles a day, and adding a half a mile a week. He had run more than 3,000 miles before undertaking the Marathon of Hope. He'd lifted weights and developed his upper body. He'd experimented with various artificial limbs, and wondered if the stump would stand up under the strain.

To finance the trip the Foxes banded together and held dances and garage sales, and Terry wrote to various businesses. More than $3,000 was raised. Esso contributed gas for the camper-van donated by the Ford Motor Company, Addidas supplied running shoes, and the Four Seasons hotels supplied accommodation. In fact, Isadore Sharp, chairman and president of Four Seasons, contributed much more. Acutely aware of the tragedy of cancer, he organized contributions from businesses from coast to coast, and in his quiet style moved various mountains to assist the run.

With the backing of the Canadian Cancer Society, with donations and with the money he and his family had raised, Terry and high school chum, Doug Alward, flew to St. John's, Newfoundland.

On the Saturday afternoon of April 12, 1980, at the St. John's waterfront, Terry dipped his artificial leg into the Atlantic Ocean.

Vancouver was 5,300 miles and six months away.

Flushed with hope, armed with spare legs and parts for the artificial leg, Terry Fox and Doug Alward drove to the waterfront in St. John's, Newfoundland. There, with only a few curious onlookers and a CBC camera crew as witnesses, Terry began his amazing run. He stopped briefly at the City Hall where Mayor Dorothy Wyatt presented him with a scroll, and had him wear the chain of office. Cancer Society president Millard Ayre had the Society's flag raised over the City Hall, and with horns blaring, Terry started off to Vancouver. The early mornings were cold and rainy; snow and high winds plagued the beginning of the trip. Often, the wind forced Doug to open the back doors of the van to form a windbreak, as Terry ran behind. It didn't work; it was too difficult to maintain the pace he'd hoped for. Nevertheless, at Come-by-Chance, ninety-three miles away, his mood was bullish. And in contrast to the inclement weather was the warmth with which he was met by the people of Newfoundland. Their good humour and generosity provided an auspicious beginning to Terry's Marathon of Hope. Earlier, he had arranged with War Amputations of Canada to service—if that's the right word—the artificial legs, and to supply new ones. The biggest problem was the artificial legs had not been designed for running, and the stump of his leg was later to blister, bleed, and develop painful sores. At one point the blood was streaming down the thin tubes that formed the lower part of the mechanical limb. He told a radio interviewer he had wanted to keep the same sock on the artificial foot until he reached Vancouver. Later, in Toronto, he referred again to the sock: "It didn't work out that way. It's worn out completely on the bottom, it's brown, it's dirty, and it stinks."

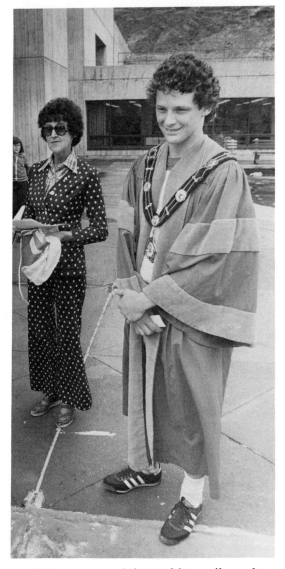

Nova Scotia was the loneliest part of the entire trip. He was doing twenty-eight to thirty miles a day at times, even though the weather was atrocious. The place Bill Vigars first met Terry was at Edmundston. Terry was wearing his baggy sweatsuit (without stripes), and black toque. There was snow, sleet, rain and wind. When the entourage could, it stayed in private homes. Otherwise, it was the smelly van, smelly from the chemical toilet and normal odour of human bodies sweating from exertion. (I'll never forget my first impression of the group. The smell. Everything smelled, the van, Terry, everything.) Frequently Terry would eliminate his noon-time nap and visit local schools, carrying his message to the children. It was in Prince Edward Island that Terry first realized that radio was the most powerful medium in getting his message through. Radio was later to play a major role across the country, said Vigars. In Halifax, Nova Scotia, brother Darrell, who obtained early graduation, joined in the cavalcade to help Terry's run (Betty, Rolly and Darrell had here the first of two reunions). His role was critical. Terry was fierce and intense while Doug was shy and reserved. Darrell became the travelling jokester, prankster and punster, keeping up spirits when the going got tough.

Near the end of the Maritime run, and serving as a hint of things to come, was the reception for Terry at Grand Falls, New Brunswick, where Cancer Society member Stan Barker had arranged a huge turnout. Each day, Cancer Society people collected and deposited the returns. It would later take scores of volunteers just to handle the thousands of cheques that poured in daily.

On June 21 he entered the province of Quebec.

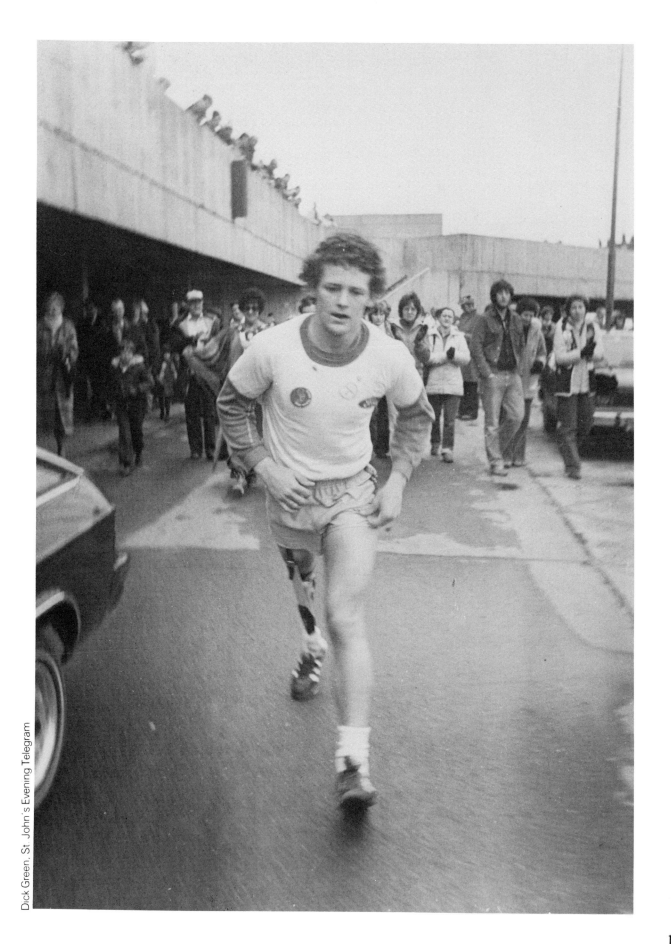

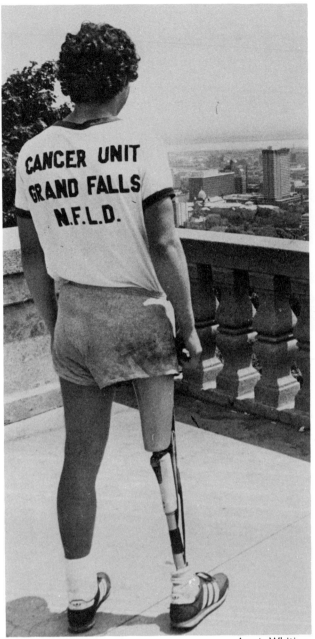

Aussie Whiting

Running along the St. Lawrence River in the province of Quebec was the most attractive part of the run, Terry said later. In Quebec City, Terry, agog with the strikingly beautiful, centuries-old architecture, quipped, "This would make a great place to play hide and seek." But if running along the shores of the St. Lawrence was the most attractive, the official response wasn't. Although people who gathered at the roadside would cheer him on, there hadn't been the advance drum-beating evident in the Maritimes. Hence the majority of the public was unaware of the magnitude of the task Terry had set for himself. But while he was down emotionally from the less-than-hoped-for response, his mental toughness remained embedded. Running into Montreal he was joined by a cadre of disabled people in wheelchairs, and former Montreal Alouette kicker Don Sweet ran into the city with him. At one point Terry cracked to Sweet, "Am I making you sweat?" Sweet and Terry later embraced (right).

Terry looks at the Montreal skyline (left).

Well-wishers, friends and critics of the run all urged Terry to consult regularly with doctors along the route. At one point the Cancer Society was criticized for "forcing him on his frantic pace." But no one was able to force Terry to do anything. He told this writer if he went to a doctor he knew what the doctor would say: ease off the pace, or take several days off a week, or stop running. None of these options existed for Terry Fox. It was seven days a week, twenty-six (or more) miles a day. Sweat pouring from his limbs, his stump frequently aching painfully, sores and cysts building from the constant punishing motion, Terry vowed the run would continue.

One day outside LaChute, Quebec, after running twenty-six miles, he stood in a phone booth for a full hour doing an open-line show on a radio station in Seattle, Washington.

(Later, during the CTV tribute to Terry Fox, the premier who most elequently expressed the feeling of the people was Rene Levesque.)

As he neared Hawkesbury on the Ontario border, he *knew* from reports that the momentum was building.

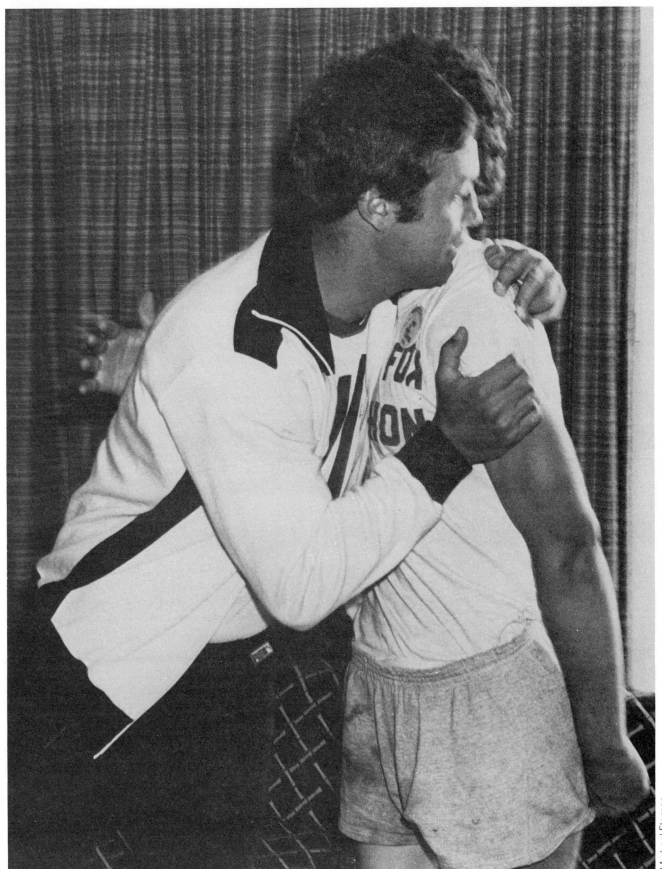

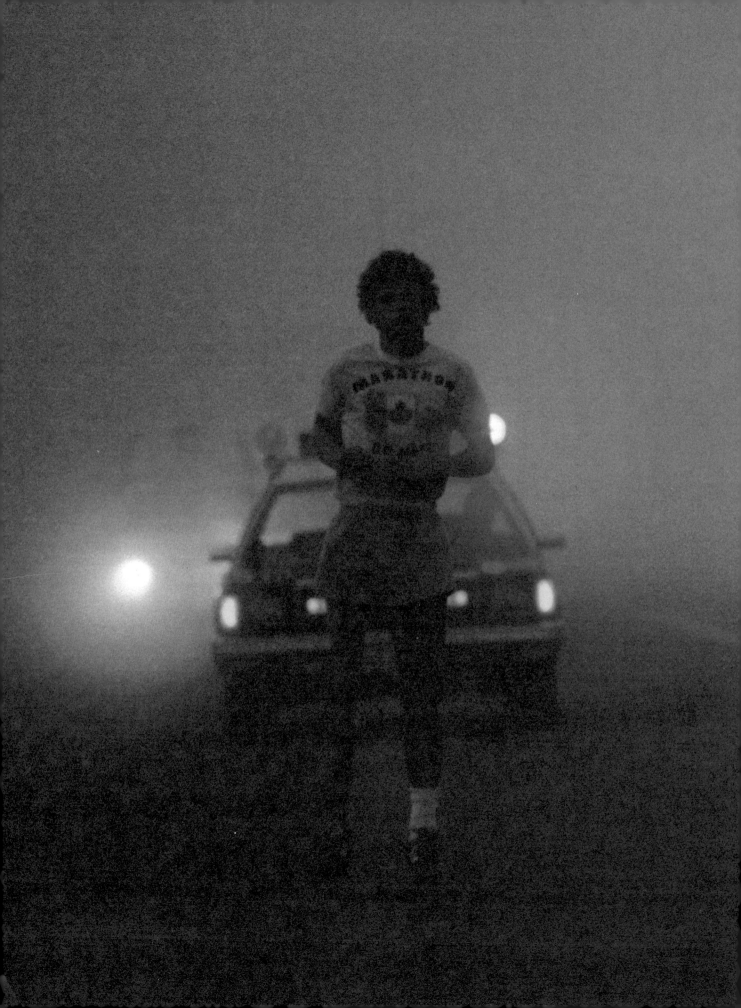

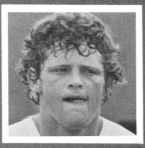
Slow down? He had to. Terry was ahead of his pace, 1,828 miles from the start, and had to run half days because Ottawa was set to receive him for the Canada Day celebrations. Ontario was a key in his raising of money for research. By now the Ontario Provincial Police had joined the cavalcade, and provided a protective cordon around the lonely runner. As he approached Ottawa, the crowds grew. Terry first met Governor General Edward Schreyer, and, later, received his largest ovation to date at the Sparks Street Mall, where he gave a stirring speech. Crowds, it seemed, buoyed his determination. They were to multiply across the province.

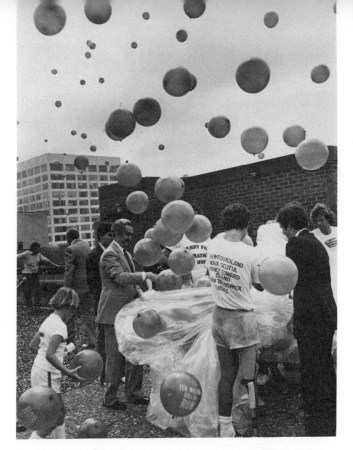

From the roof of the Ottawa Four Seasons hotel, Terry and Jean Luc Pepin, federal minister of transport, released 1,000 balloons (right), all carrying Terry's message. Moments later, two young cyclists, Garth Walker and Jim Brown (below), arrived after a twenty-four hour bike race from Toronto, bringing thousands of dollars in cash and pledges and a huge scroll with autographs of well-wishers from Toronto. The cyclists had ridden throughout the night, through thunderstorms and menacing traffic. Walker and Brown, like many touched by Terry, continued their fund-raising efforts thereafter.

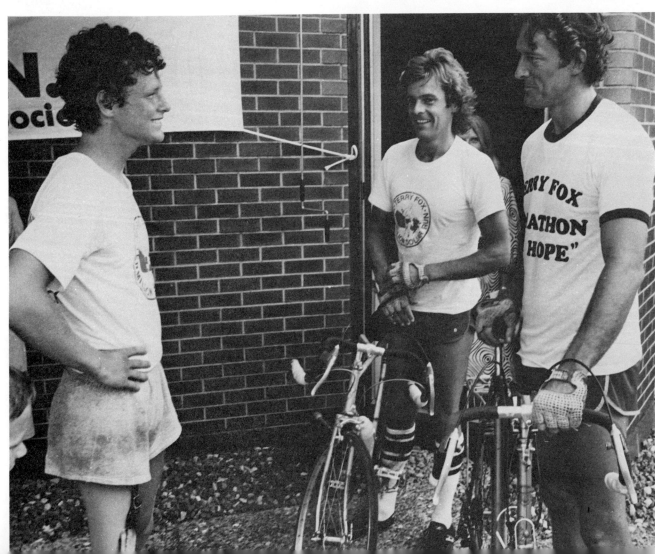

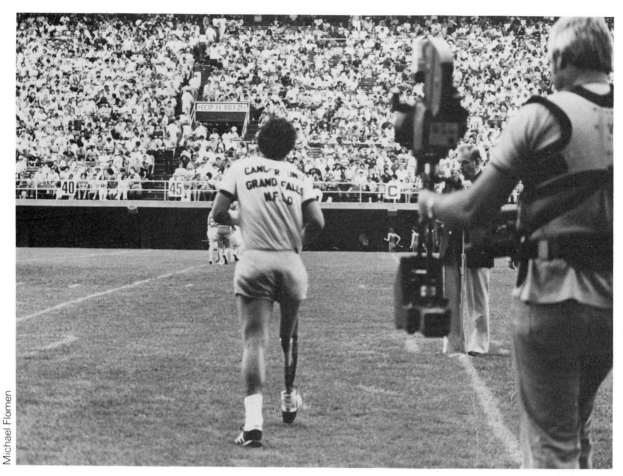

Michael Flomen

The night of his arrival in Ottawa, Terry dined with Ron Foxx, linebacker for the Ottawa Rough Riders and a dozen volunteers from the local division of the Cancer Society. The next afternoon he was invited to perform the ceremonial kickoff at a game between the Ottawa Rough Riders and the Saskatchewan Roughriders at Lansdowne Stadium. Here Bill Vigars picks up the story:

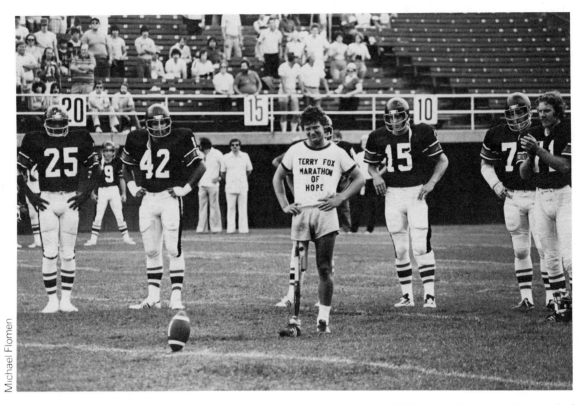

Michael Flomen

"The first really big impact of the run was the kickoff at the game. We were down underneath the stands (We had to walk in—a security guard would not let us park the van nearby). Terry tried to work out how to kick the ball, afraid he might slip on the artificial turf. First he tried kicking with the artificial leg. The ball rolled about five feet, and he realized he would have to balance on the artificial leg and kick with his real leg. We practiced a couple of times and then started walking up the stairs to the field. Terry said, 'I don't know if I should do this.' I thought to myself, wouldn't it be nice if they gave him a real round of applause. As the announcer said, 'Ladies and gentlemen . . .' the crowd saw Terry walking to the sidelines; they rose and gave him a fantastic ovation. It brought tears to my eyes." At centrefield, Terry balanced on the artificial leg, and sent the ball over the head of the player waiting to catch it (opposite). He watched later as Saskatchewan defeated Ottawa. Just before the end of the game, he slipped off to the hotel, exhausted but elated.

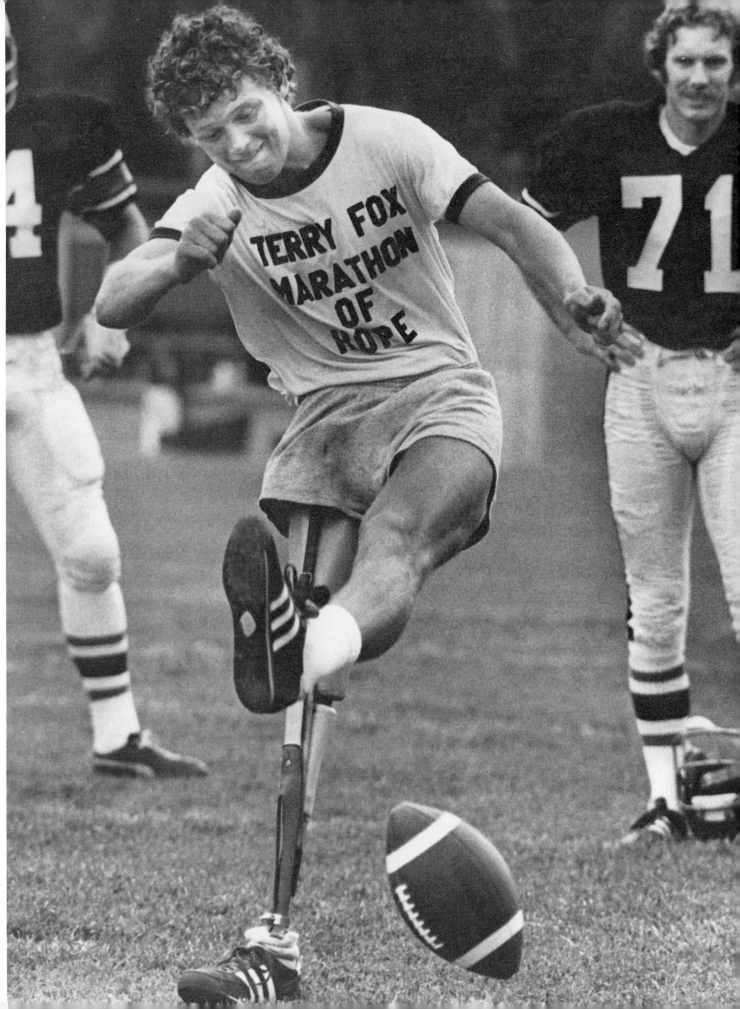

A poorly-briefed prime minister (he didn't know Terry was running to raise funds for cancer research), nonetheless received Terry (right). Terry later said bluntly, "It wasn't what I'd hoped it would be . . . but he's a really nice man and it was great meeting him."

Below, in a rare moment of repose, brother Darrell, Terry and Doug Alward rest before resuming the run. At right, Terry ties his shoe, prior to setting out for Toronto.

Overleaf, Jack Lambert, a Cancer Society official and later to become a close friend of Terry, is seen picking up donations on the long road from Ottawa.

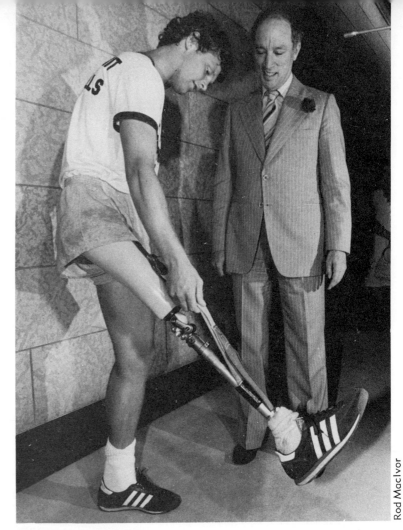

Rod MacIvor

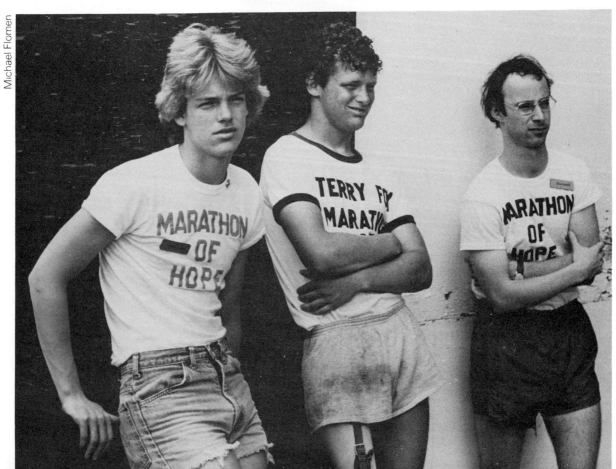

Michael Flomen

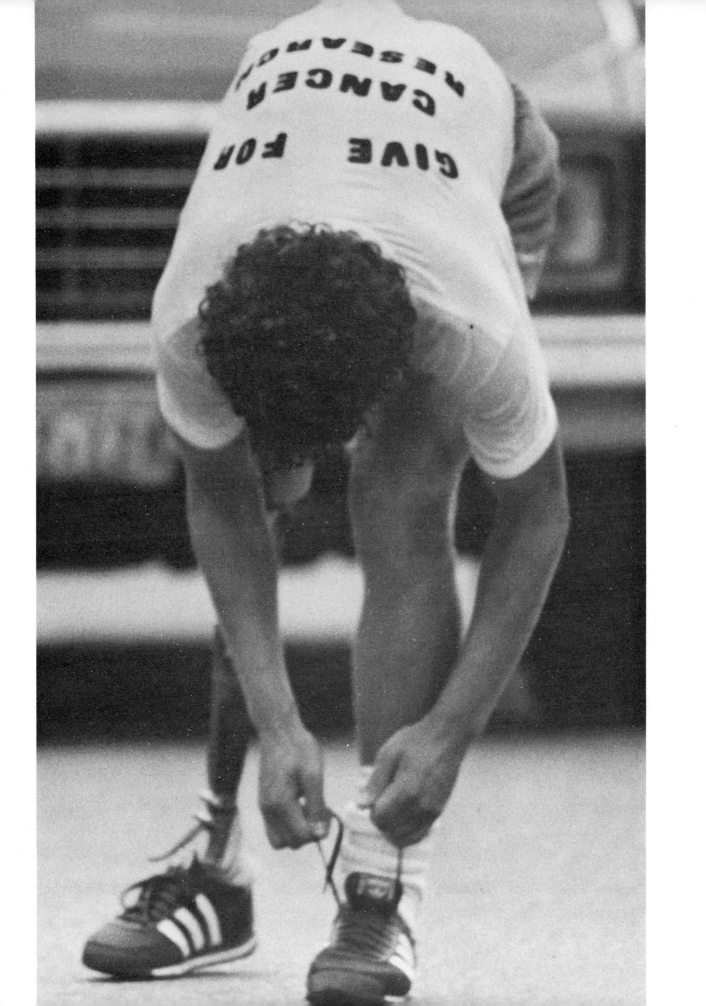

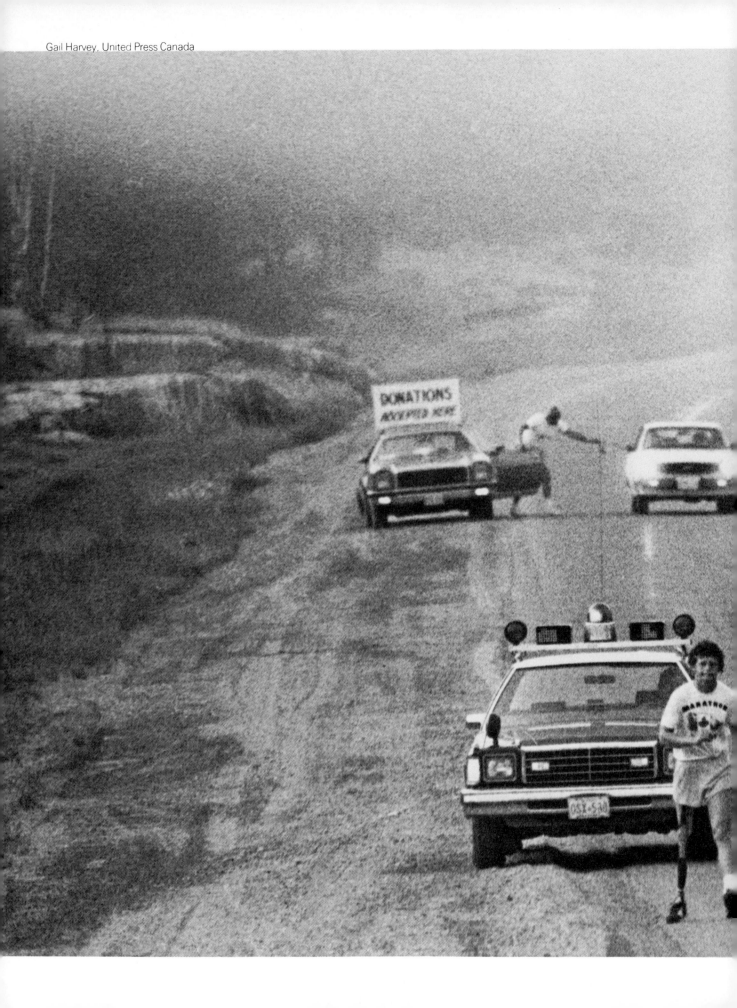

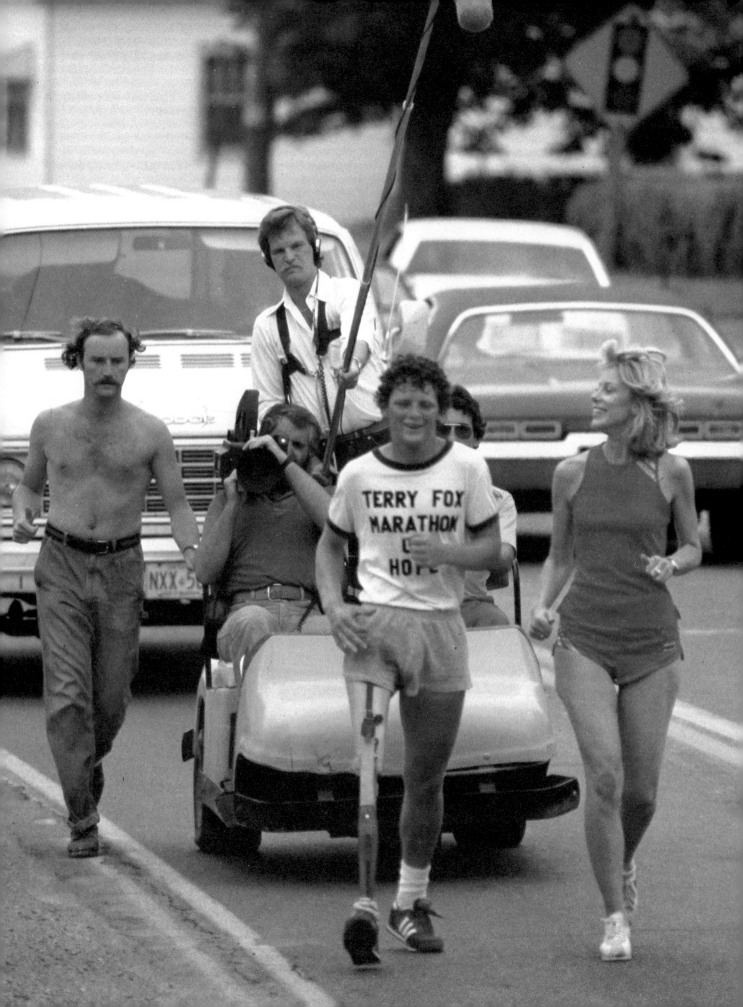

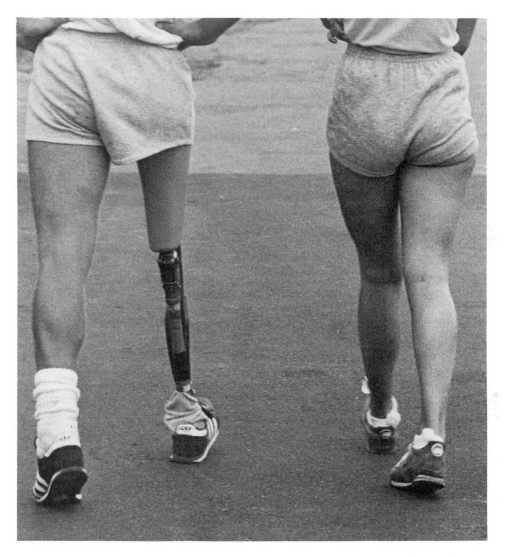

Outside Bowmanville, east of Toronto, a crew from NBC's Real People TV series caught up with Terry. Host Sarah Purcell (left) ran with him, and then, as Terry said later, "asked a lot of good questions."

By this time in the run, Terry had raised international interest, and telephone queries were coming in from Great Britain and Europe, and as far away as Japan. ABC's Good Morning America program later tried to film him, and the wire services kept filing regular stories. With little chance to relax, Terry stole the odd moment (above) with visitors who kept reappearing on the run. One such occasion, and one of the most touching moments in the marathon occurred near Medoc, Ontario. A woman with a six-year-old boy approached Terry. "My son has cancer," she said. "Terry, you're running for my little boy."

Nearing Toronto, the most dramatic events were yet to happen. Toronto had planned a major welcome and celebration.

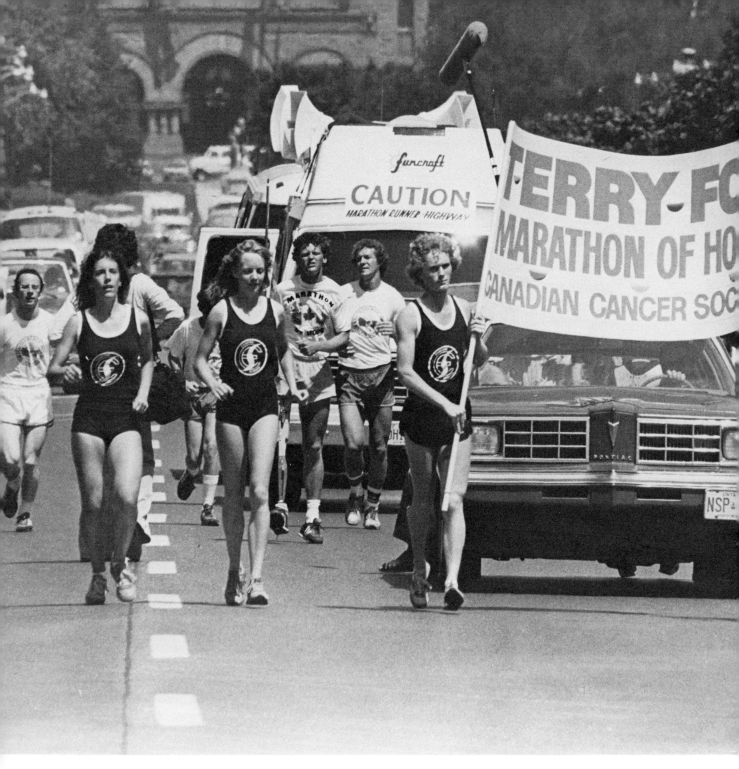

July 11, 1980. 11.30 a.m.

Flanked by one of his heroes, Darryl Sittler, as well as by brothers Fred and Darrell, sister Judy, and with parents in a van behind, Terry took University Avenue by storm. Thousands lined the streets as he ran in the blistering 30°C heat. The day before, the *Toronto Star* had flown in the Fox family, a surprise for Terry.

That morning, on the early run into Metro Toronto, he'd stopped at Scarborough Town Hall. In the arching interior 3,000 people wouldn't stop applauding. A tiny, blonde cancer victim, after her brief speech, gave Terry a donation, bringing him to tears.

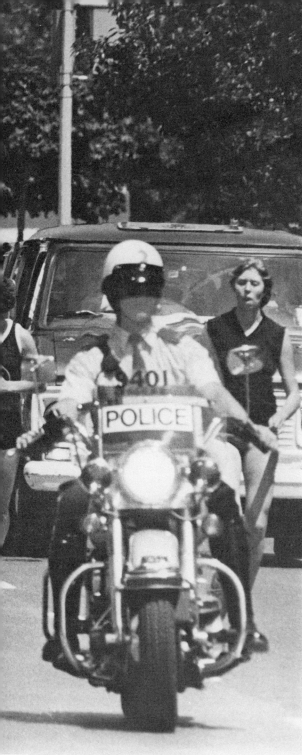

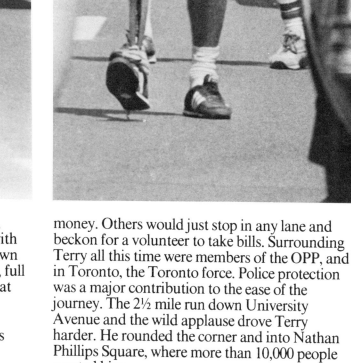

Along Terry's run to Nathan Phillips Square, scores of volunteers could scarcely keep up with the cash thrown at them. Volunteer Karl Brown said one American tourist emptied his wallet, full of $50 bills into his bag after taking one look at Terry.

Watching the phenomenon that morning was awesome. In the middle of traffic cars would squeal to a stop, the occupants holding out money. Others would just stop in any lane and beckon for a volunteer to take bills. Surrounding Terry all this time were members of the OPP, and in Toronto, the Toronto force. Police protection was a major contribution to the ease of the journey. The 2½ mile run down University Avenue and the wild applause drove Terry harder. He rounded the corner and into Nathan Phillips Square, where more than 10,000 people greeted him.

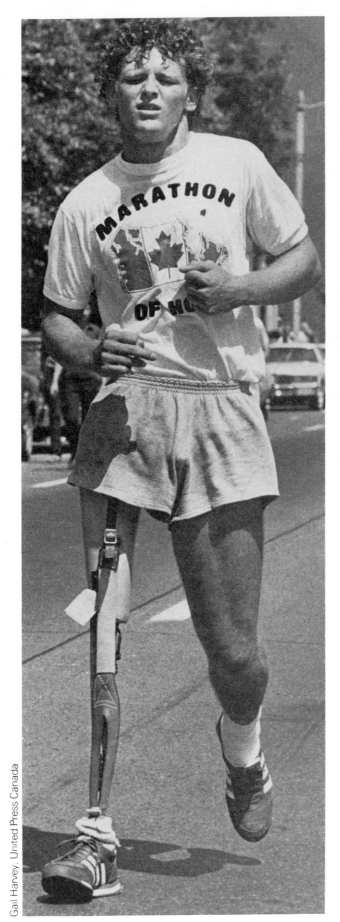
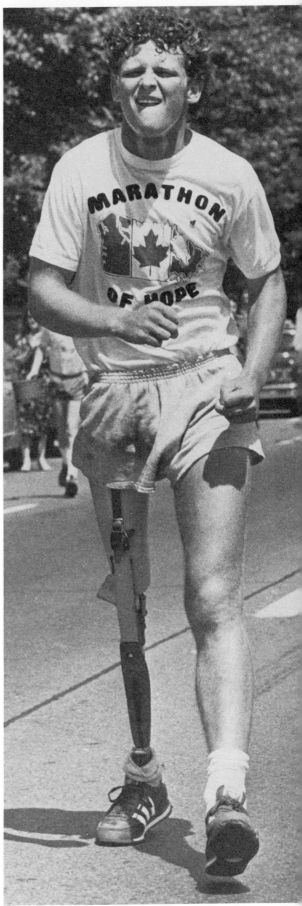

Gail Harvey, United Press Canada

32

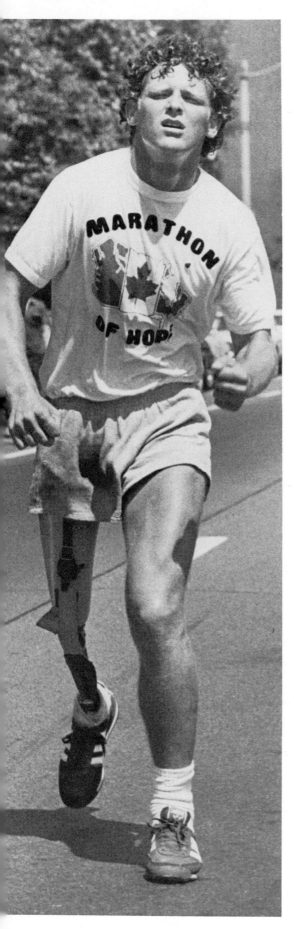

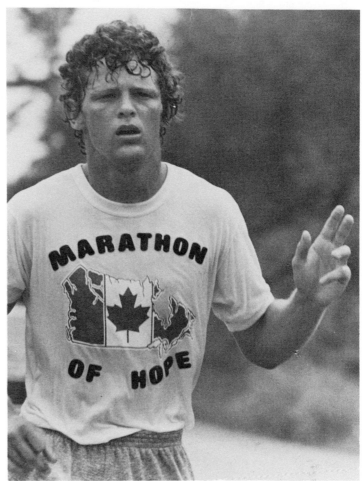

Gail Harvey in these photographs captures the essence of Terry's agony as he pounded along the pavement, each step no easier than the last, each exertion as taxing as the next. Terry is seen wearing his favourite T-shirt, two of which were given to him by a woman in Marmora. She would later deliver a dozen more. Of all the hundreds of T-shirts offered to him along the route, the one shown is the one he wore thereafter. He eschewed any T-shirt with a commercial message, nor would he allow any use of his name or cause for commercial purposes. "I'm not going to make a cent out of this," he told this writer, "not now and not later." It was the integrity of his purpose that made the most lasting impact.

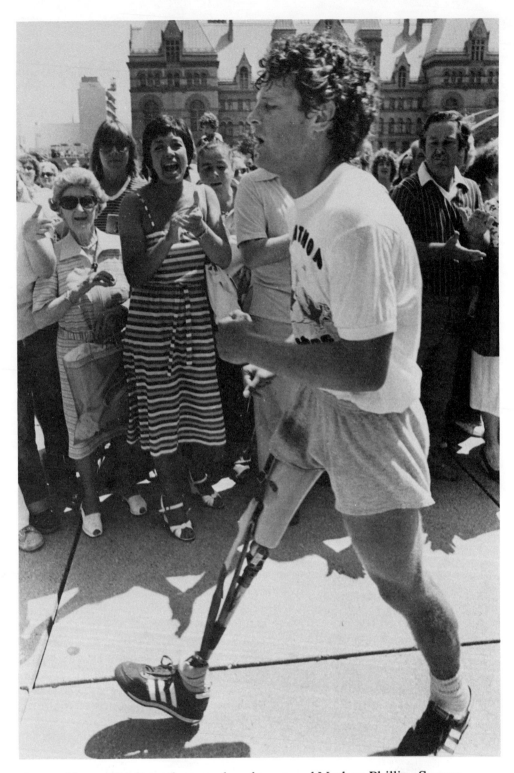

Joy and love came from the crowds as he entered Nathan Phillips Square (above). The cheering built as he approached the bandstand. Soon after, draped in a prize possession—Darryl Sittler's famous number 27 hockey sweater (right)—Terry told of his crusade for funds for cancer research, his sole and compelling message.

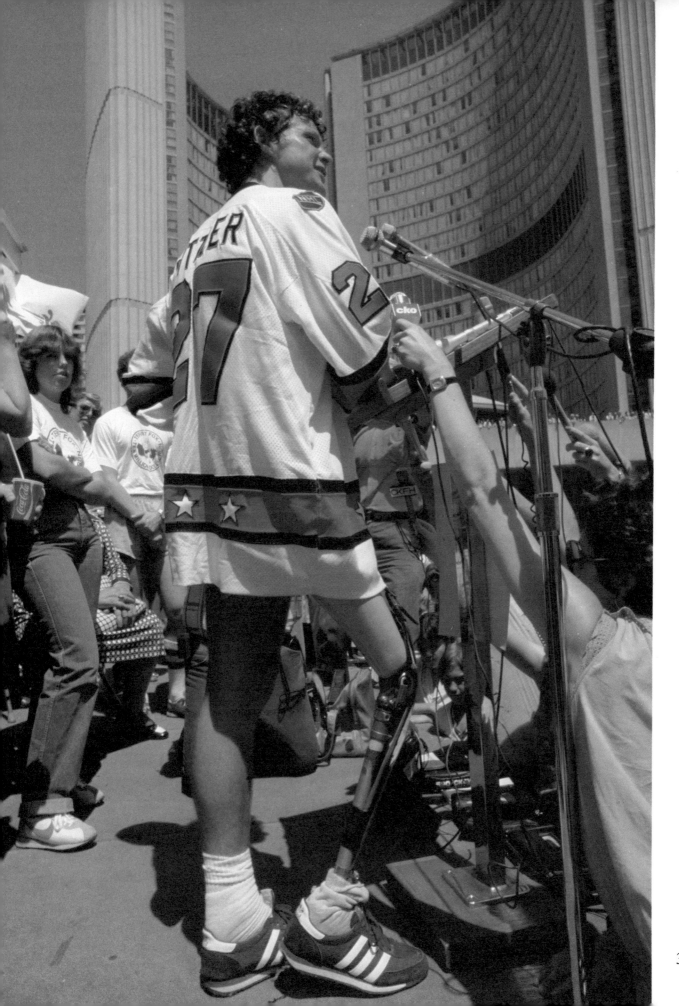

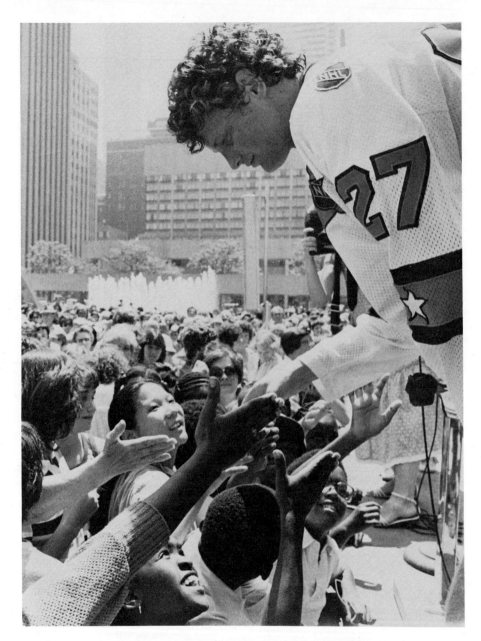

There were seemingly endless speeches, mostly from politicians, but television star Al Waxman, honorary chairman of the Canadian Cancer Society, kept the dignitaries moving as swiftly as possible. After all the speeches, the crowds pressed forward to grasp Terry's hand (above), seeking autographs, wishing him well. Terry Fox had cut right through to all the people. Then, framed by huge policemen (right), Terry continued a whirlwind of activity; another press conference, an interview, a fitting for yet another artificial leg—and then, some fun. The family went secretly to the CN Tower, saw the sights, played pinball and bumper car (where his artificial leg came off after a crash).

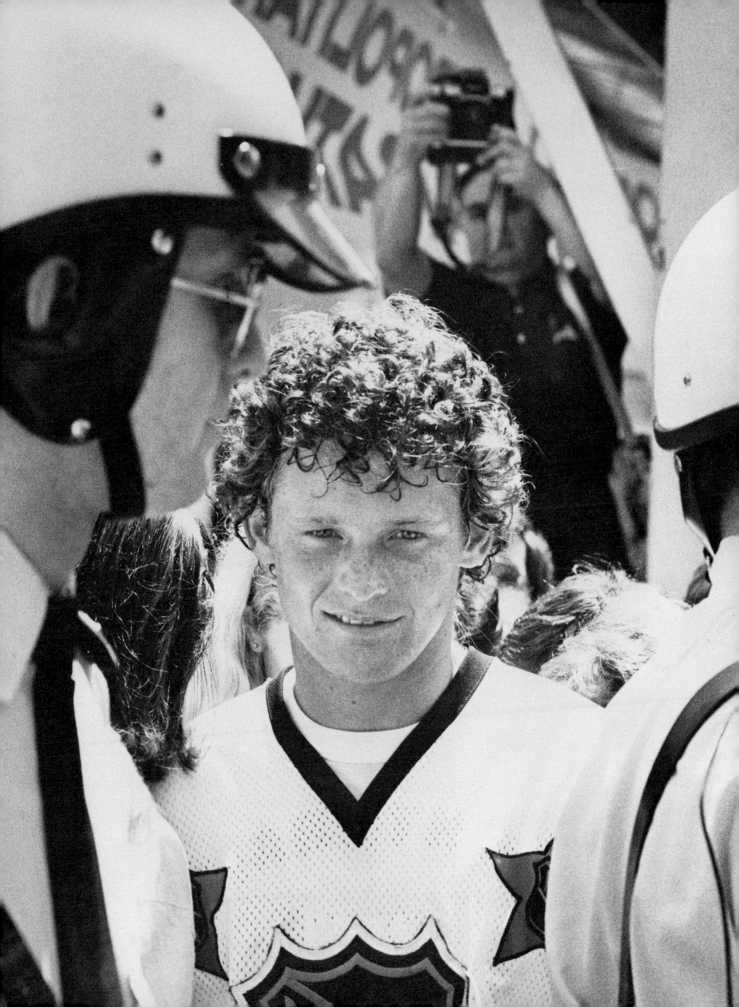

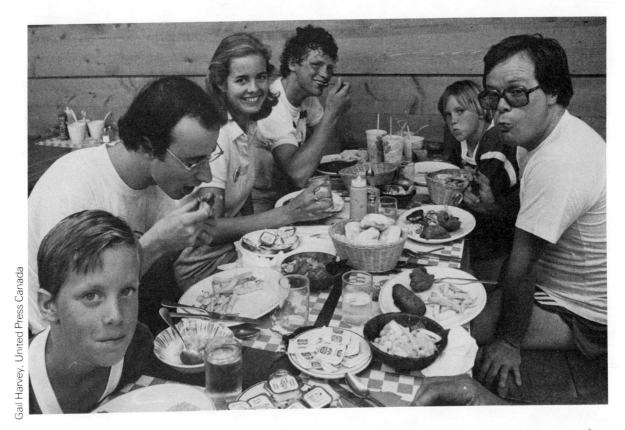

Terry had been up since 4.15 a.m., but it was time for yet another function. With the mascot for the Toronto Blue Jays, Terry talks to a player before preparing for the ceremonial pitch. Pitching is easier than kicking a football, and the pictures overleaf show his technique.

After the game, he went to his suite at the Four Seasons Yorkville. It had been the most taxing day of the entire run, and Terry was still elated with the reception he'd received.

On normal days, Terry would get to bed about 8.30 p.m., and the only time to relax and have fun was at dinner. There were frequent food fights, but the group established one rule. "We couldn't get the restaurant dirty, and if a guy was hitting you with food, you had to sit still." Once, at Barrie, Ontario, Darrell saturated Bill Vigars with soya sauce, and in return suffered an attack of plum sauce. But it wasn't all fun each evening. Sometimes, when the pressures were too great, there would be an odd angry exchange, or one member wouldn't speak to another for a day. But the troupe held together through every difficulty.

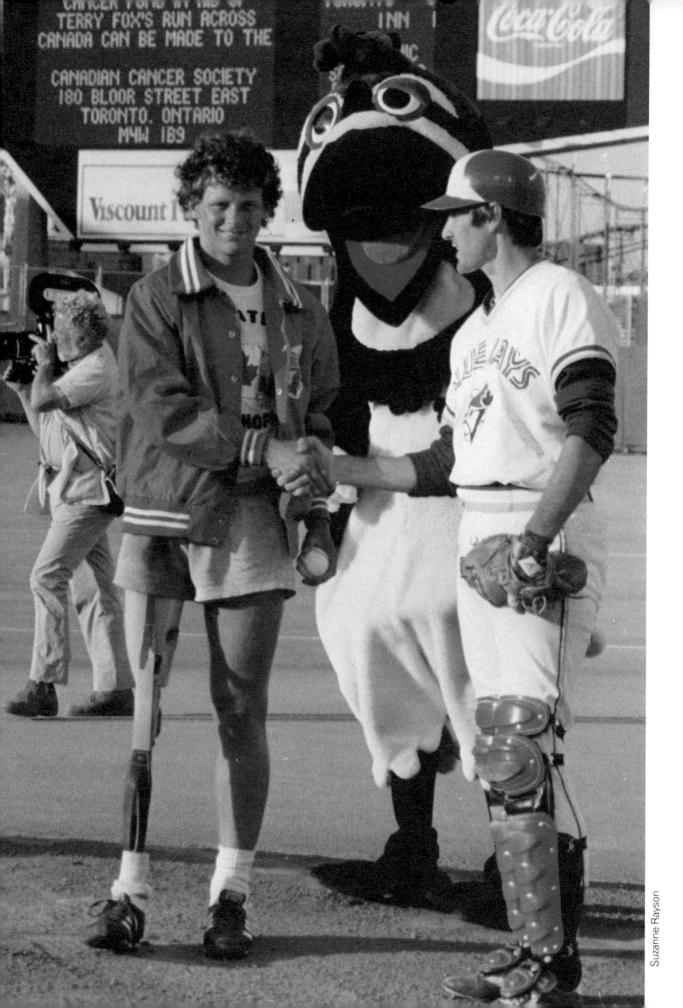

39

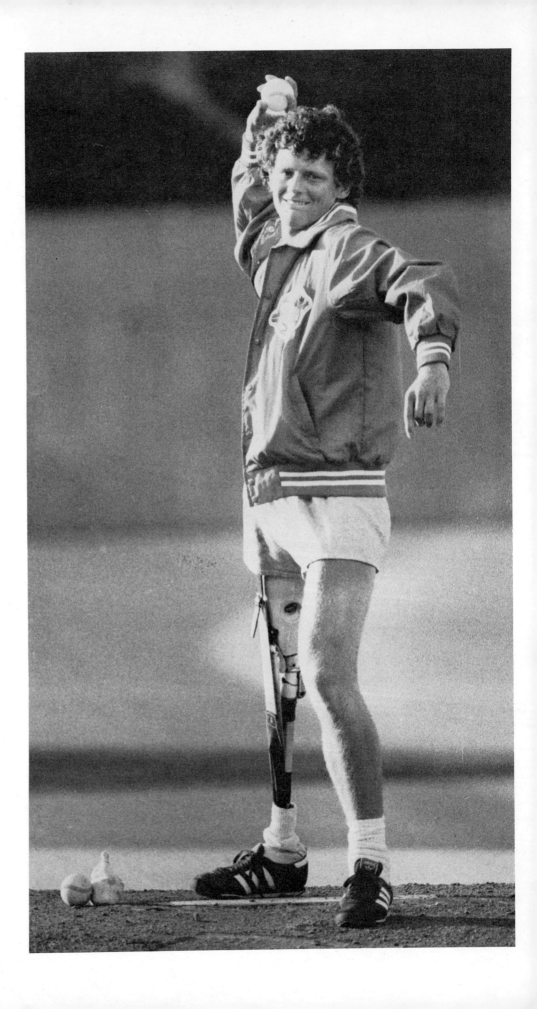

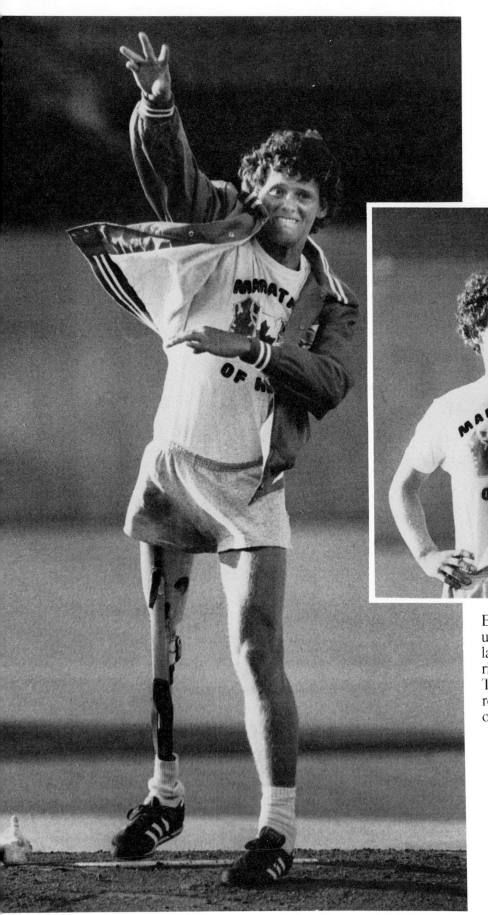

Ever the athlete, Terry winds
up and delivers a hard pitch to
launch the game. Despite the
rigors of that exhausting day in
Toronto, Terry (above)
responds to the standing
ovation at Exhibition Stadium.

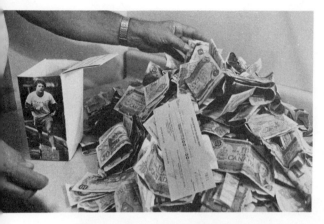

The money continued to pour in as they left Toronto. Jack Lambert counted out $3,000 (left) from one event, and, by the time they had reached a major highway (still inside Toronto), they had gathered $8,000. While Terry ran straight ahead, Darrell (below) spent the marathon zigging and zagging as motorists honked to donate.

One of the classic photographs of the run (right) was taken by *Oakville Journal Record* photographer Pete Martin, as Terry ran in the early hours of the morning. Terry's 'mental toughness' was monumental; the inside jokes and the run were incidental to the daily goal: twenty-six miles or more per day, seven days a week.

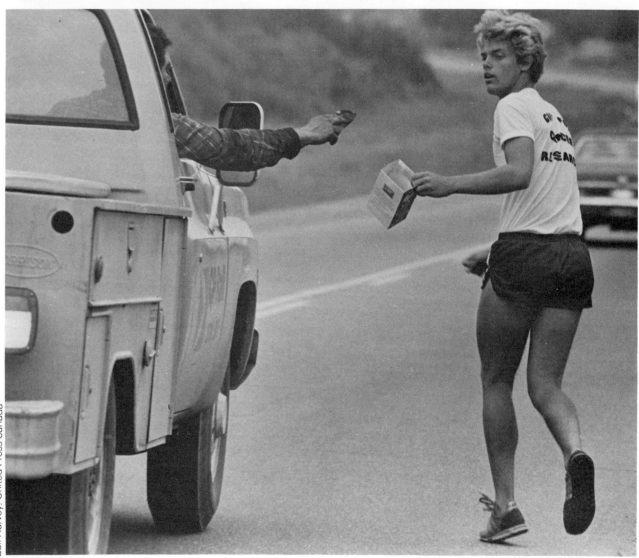

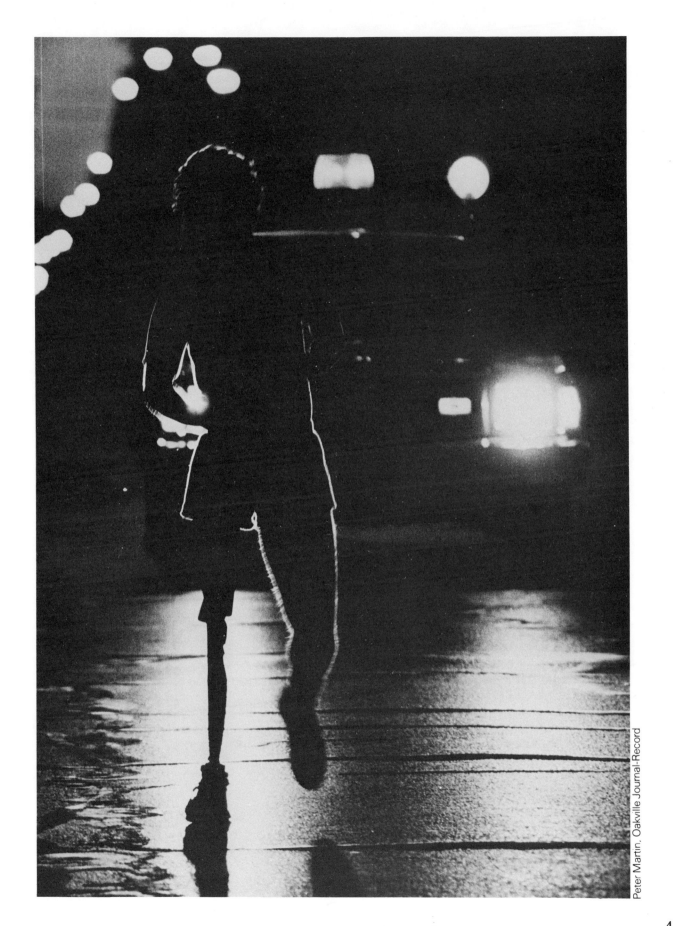

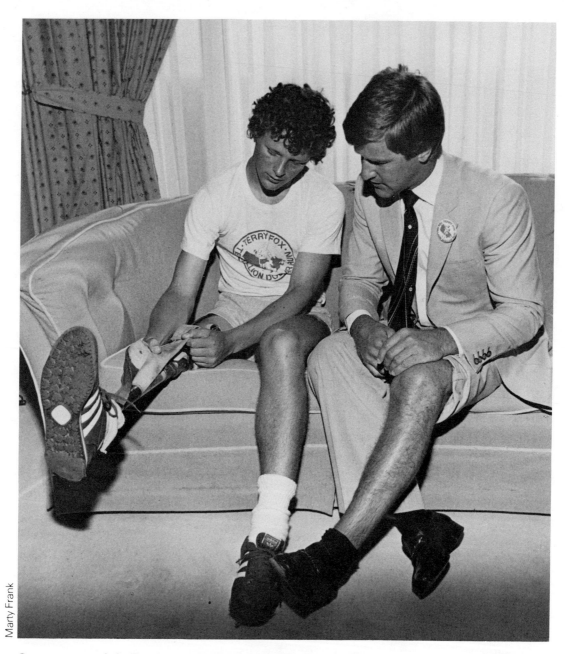

Marty Frank

One superstar left. Terry wanted to meet Bobby Orr, once described as the greatest hockey player in the world. Orr flew in and Terry came back to Toronto. Orr showed Terry his much-operated-on knee, while Terry displayed his mechanical knee. After a press conference, there was a private dinner. Orr was summoned for a flight, but retorted, "Get the next one, I want to stay here." Orr's sponsor donated $25,000—with a further $25,000 to come.

Then, once again, it was back on the road (right).

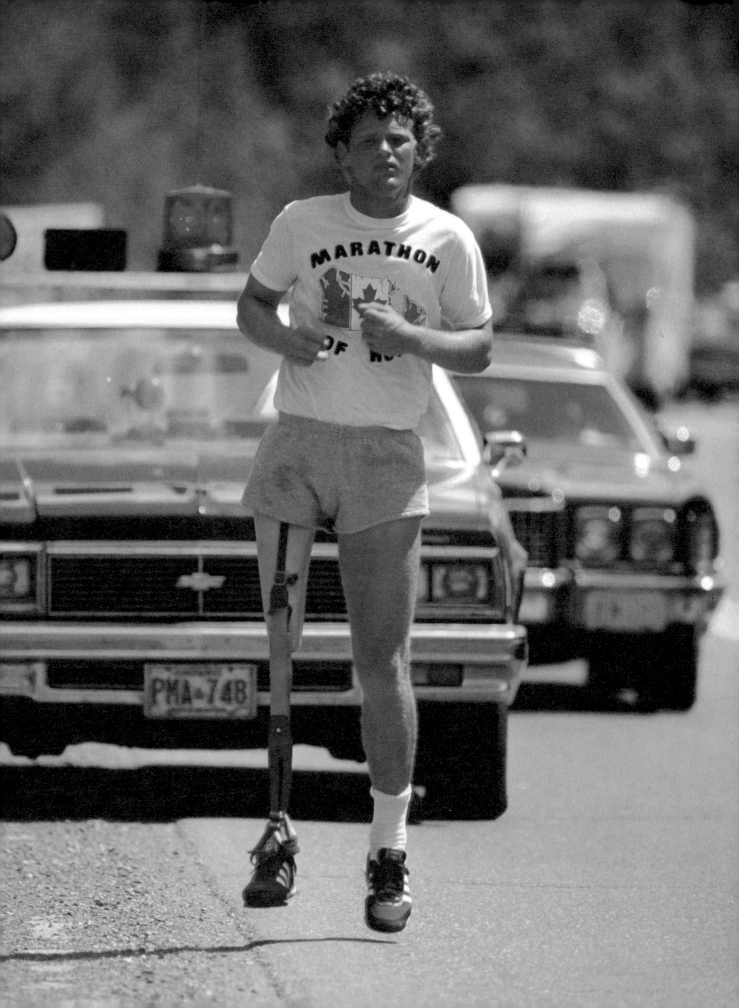

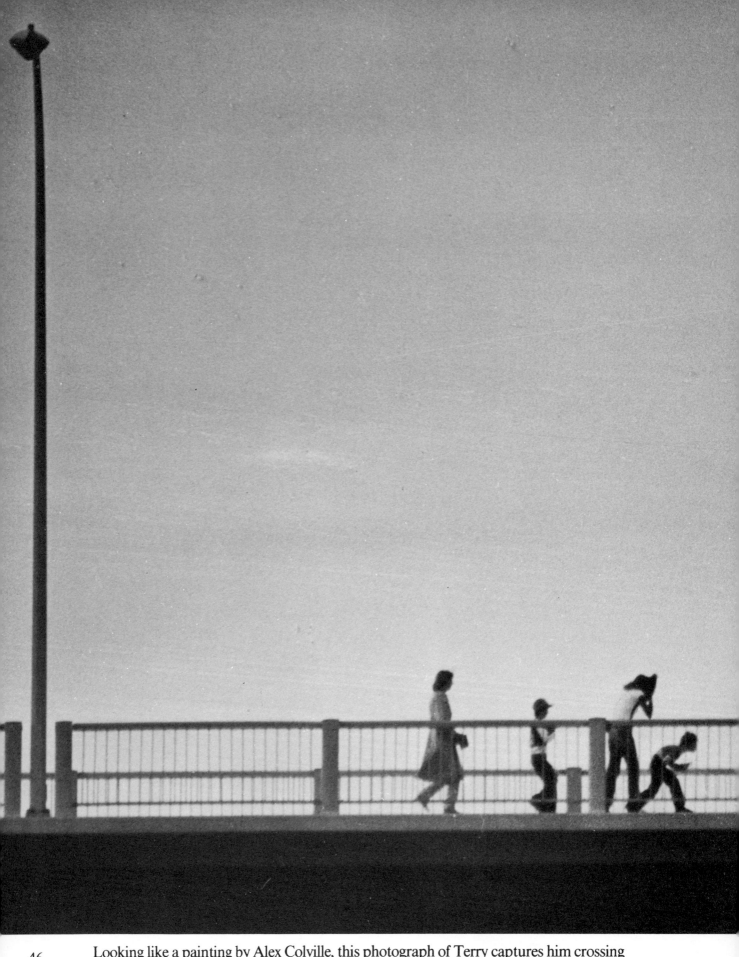

46 Looking like a painting by Alex Colville, this photograph of Terry captures him crossing
a bridge, closely followed by the curious and the admiring.

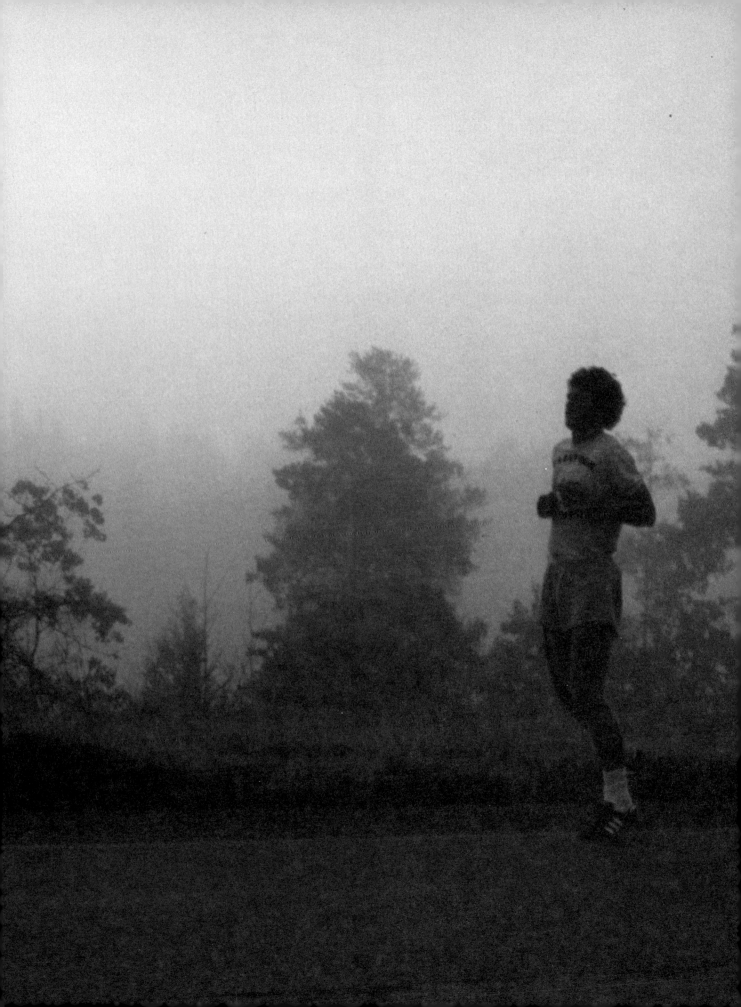

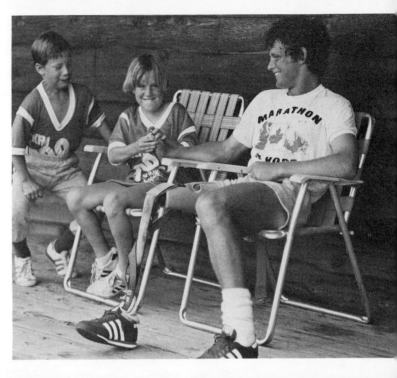

Moments of pleasure and relaxation were rare and treasured. Here, in Northern Ontario just south of Sudbury, Terry indulges in some horseplay with Kerry Anne, nine, and Patrick Vigars, eight, near the French River Trading Post. He had just completed his twenty-six miles. The youngsters accompanied Terry on part of the trip, helping with the collecting as well as some of the routine, daily chores.

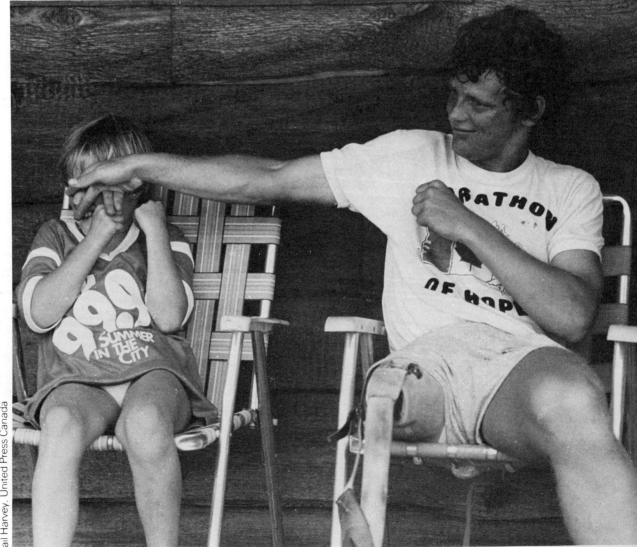

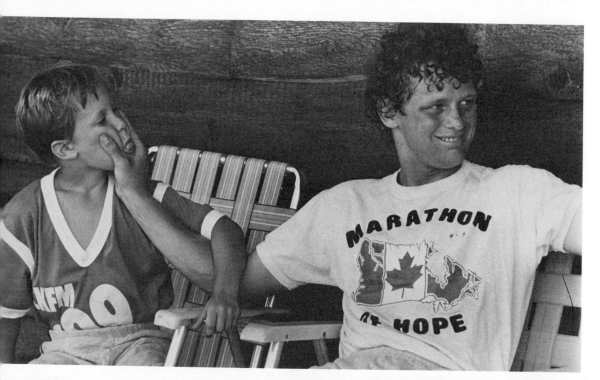

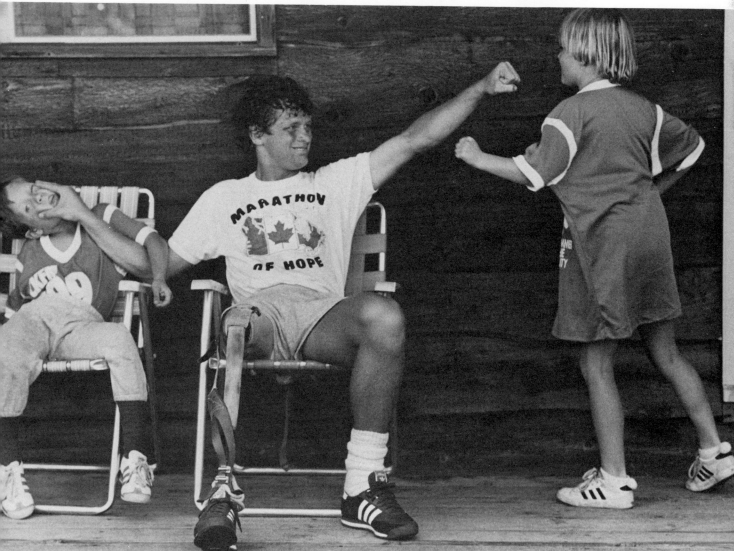

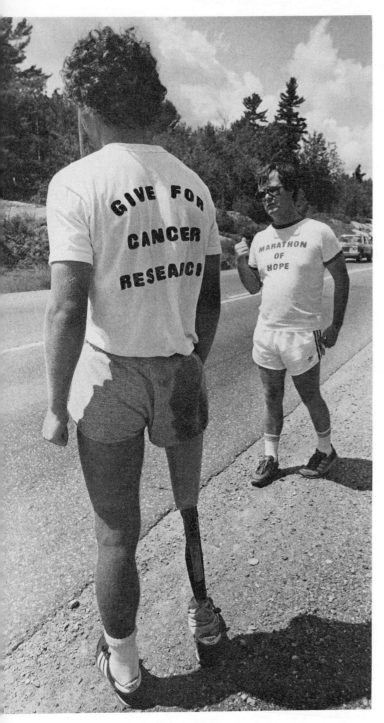

While Bill Vigars (left), who in a different context might be called a tour manager, oversaw the broad plan, it was the various district directors of the Cancer Society who handled the local receptions in their areas. Jack Lambert (right) was one who formed a close, personal bond with the runner. When Lambert handed Terry over to the next director, there were tears and embraces. As the run through Ontario north of Barrie developed, sporadic reports appeared that Terry was sick, that his amputated stump was bleeding and sore, and that he should abandon the run. Genuine concern was expressed by members of the War Amputations organization who supplied him with a number of artificial legs (at $2,000 each), and who examined the stump. Armand Viau, a prosthetist, or specialist in artificial parts, suggested body tissue could not stand the abuse of the constant pounding. He worried about the stump changing shape, the cysts and sores, the chafing, and most importantly, the flow of blood to the truncated limb. But Terry, although not distrustful of medical people (one of the drugs used for his initial chemotherapy had been developed only two years prior to his first attack), expressed reluctance to this writer about seeing doctors who might dissuade him from continuing. "His sores and his wounds healed almost every night," said Vigars. "It was impossible to make him stop . . . Terry's birthday for example, on July 28. I said, 'Listen, it's your birthday, why don't you break early today.' And Terry responded, 'The best birthday present I can give myself is to run twenty-six miles!' And he did!"

At Gravenhurst, more than 3,000 people turned out to the town's arena, gave him a huge cake and thousands of dollars. (He also received some ribald presents from his entourage.)

The weather in July and August in Ontario was hot. An occasional rain storm would sweep the route, but it was the heat that became the biggest burden. "We'd try to talk him into running, say, only twenty miles a day," Vigars said. "It was impossible to get him to stop. He took one day off in Montreal so that he hit the Ontario border on time, and he was angry about that."

Even on the hottest days he wouldn't slow down. The decisions were all Terry's. "You never made a decision without checking with Terry because it was simply *his* run."

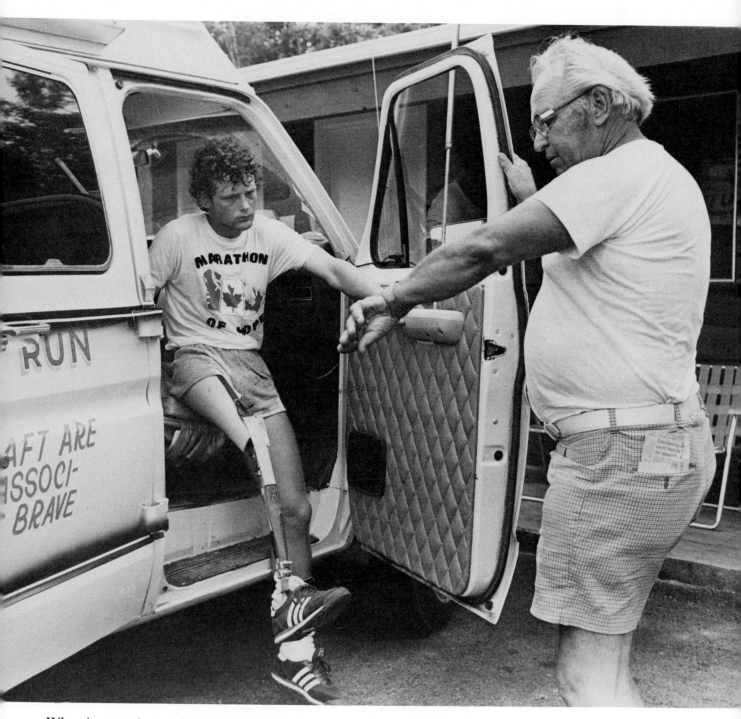

When it came time to finish a day's run, and look for a motel, Terry would always want to go back, not ahead. He'd want to see the countryside upcoming for the first time while he was running, and not from a car.

The angriest he ever became was when a columnist in B.C. wrote that Terry had run 150 miles in Quebec, then driven the rest of the way. Raging, he ordered Vigars to get the columnist on the phone instantly. From an old, hand-crank phone Terry said, "All the pain and suffering and sweat that I've put into this is worthless if you don't believe . . . if there's *one* person . . . who doesn't believe I went the whole way." A retraction appeared.

In fact, at the end of each block of running, Terry would make a mental note of some object, a sign, a lamppost, and he'd touch that same object when he resumed running. Of the 3,339 miles he covered, he *ran* every inch of the way.

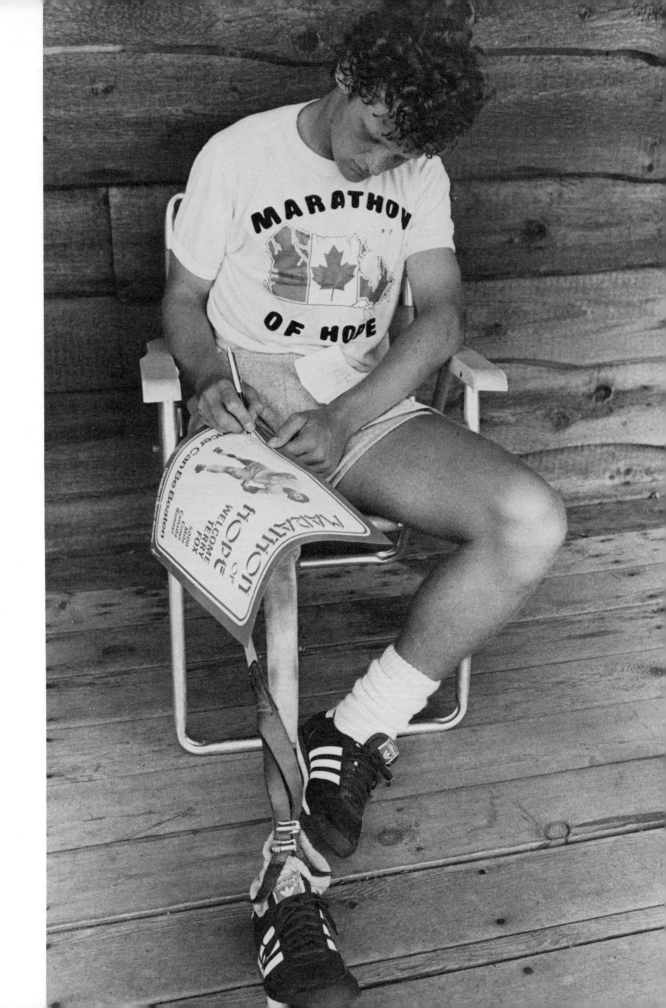

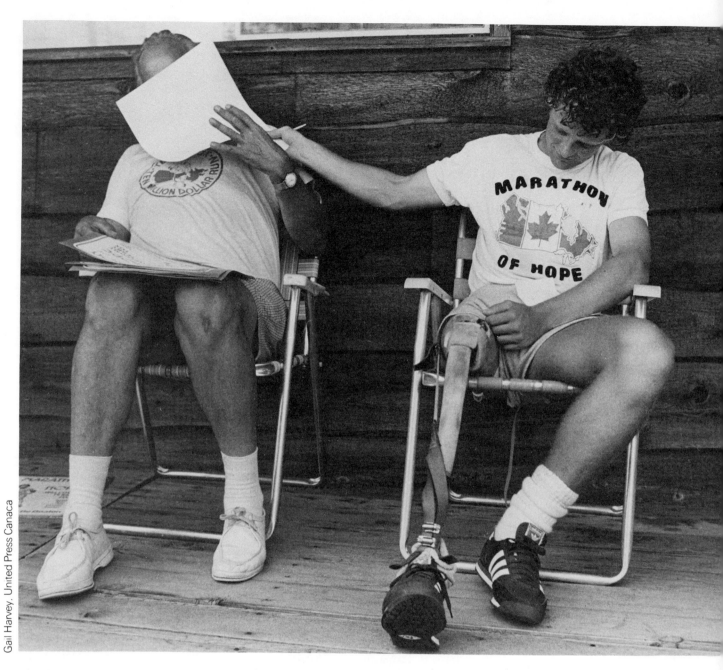

Signing autographs—everybody it seems wanted his
autograph—became easy. Terry would only have to rest the poster
on his artificial limb to provide an instant table. Terry would sign
posters, then fling them to the patient Jack Lambert (above),
who would then disperse them to the onlookers. The horseplay
during breaks broke the tension of the run.

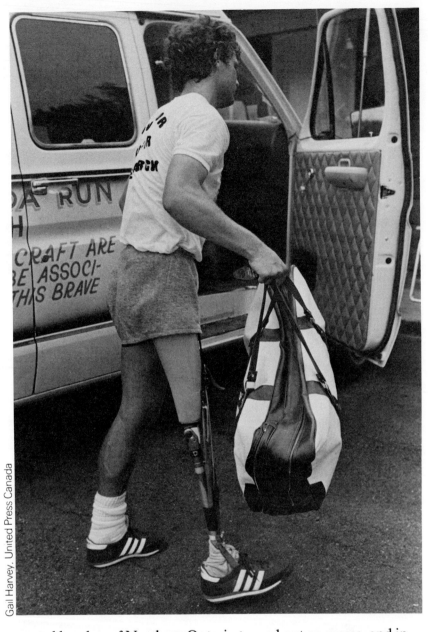

Gail Harvey, United Press Canada

People of the little towns and hamlets of Northern Ontario turned out en masse, and in almost each case the dollar sum raised vastly exceeded the total population. At the end of the day's run Terry would take his green and white Addidas bag (above), containing most of his worldly possessions, and go to a motel. At the French River Trading Post (right), Terry showered, and prepared for the inevitable local reception, followed by a private dinner. At one such dinner an onlooker shouted, "Hey . . . there's Terry Fox." Darrell, Doug, Bill and Terry eyed each other. Then—as in the TV show, *To Tell The Truth*, —each made a hesitant attempt to rise.

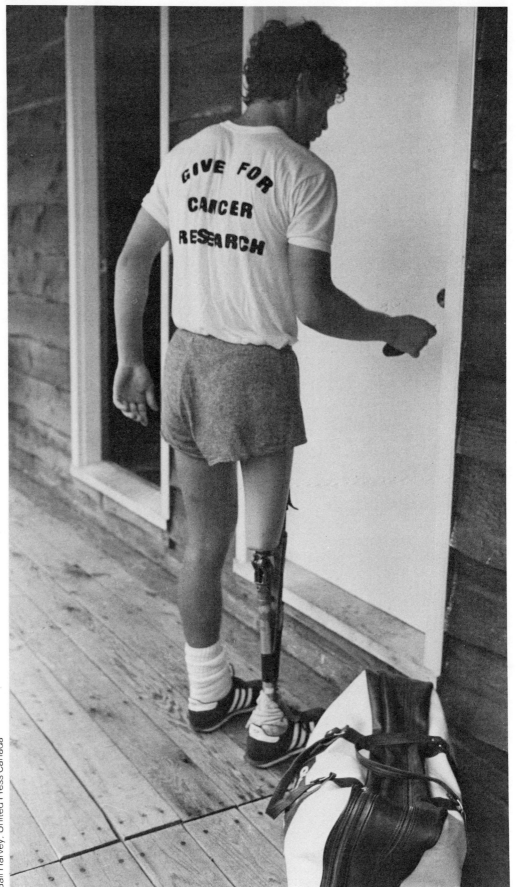

Gail Harvey, United Press Canada

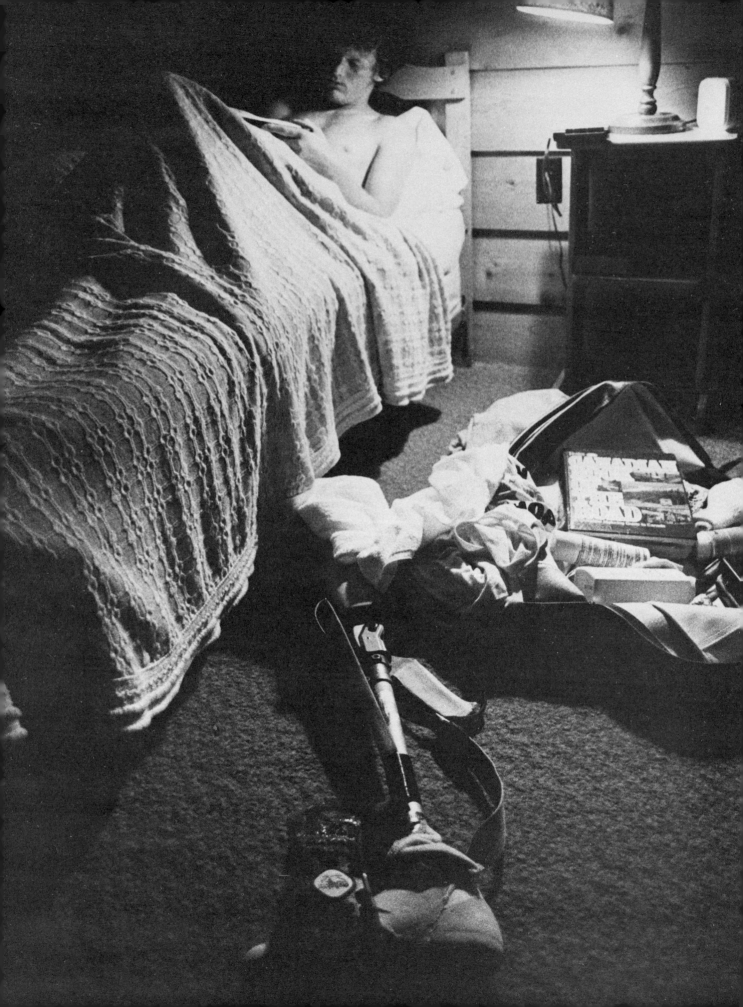

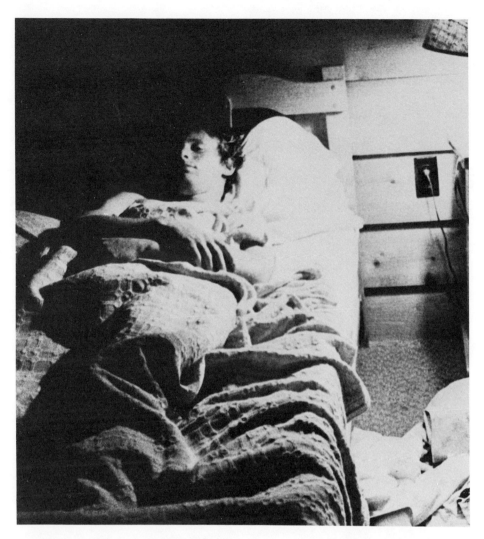

In this rare series of photographs, Terry has retired for the night and is writing in his journal, a private diary of thoughts and impressions, as well as a record of the run. Up to Thunder Bay, no one had seen the journal. Following this he would read about the next city or town in the *Canadian Road Atlas* to prepare for the upcoming day.

Then, blessed sleep.

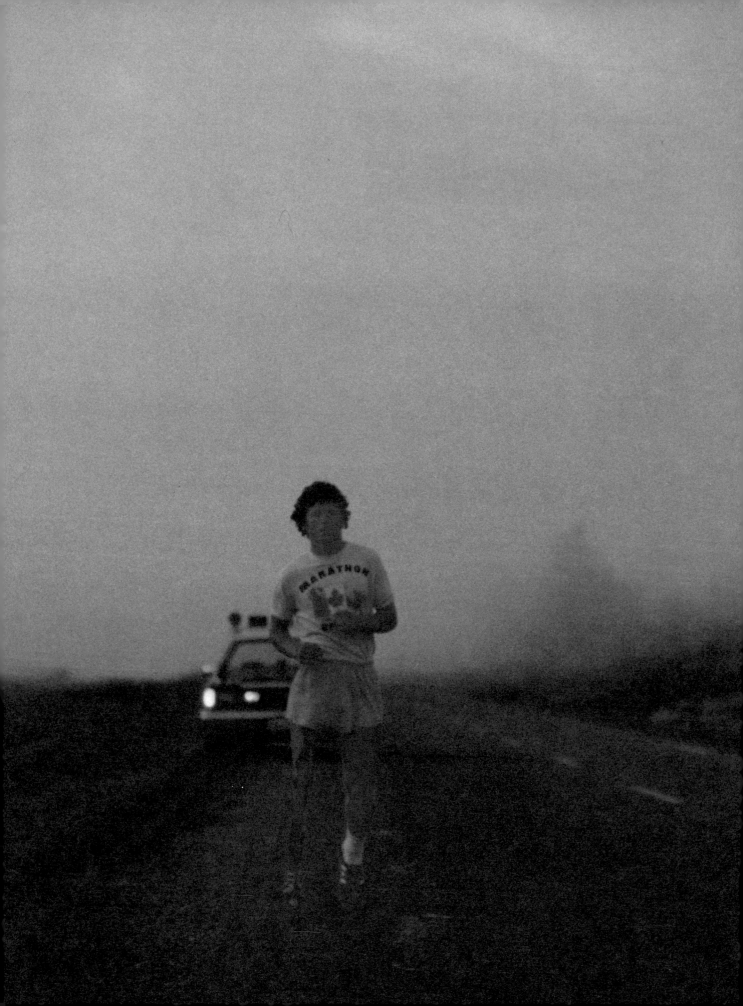

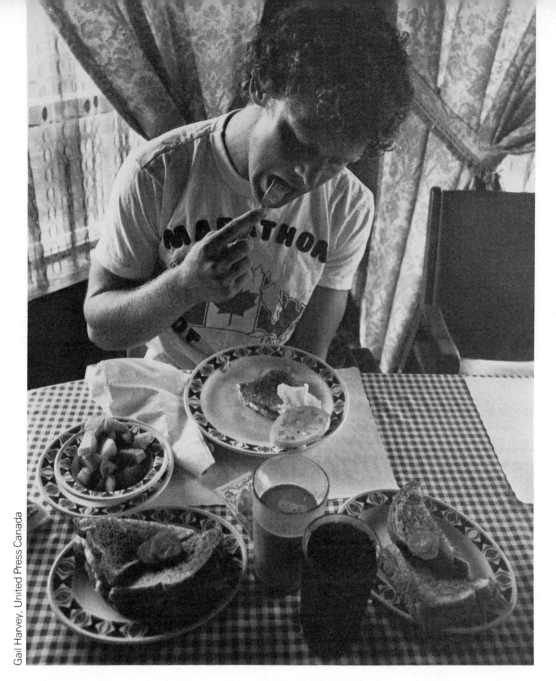

Off in the early morning, Terry covered his usual twelve miles (left) before breakfast. Some nutritionists shuddered at his diet. The rate at which he consumed so-called junk food was astonishing. At this breakfast (above), Terry had two grilled cheese sandwiches, pancakes, french fries and gravy, a chocolate milkshake and a coke. His favourite foods were pineapple, pizza, beans, rice, and peanut butter and jelly sandwiches. There was some method to this gastronomic madness. Terry studied carefully the needs of long-distance runners, and concluded that 'carbohydrate loading' was needed to replenish the body and prepare for the next day.

At dinner, Terry would sometimes startle the waitress by ordering *everything* on the menu. Doug would order nothing, knowing that something would be left over.

Overleaf: After a nap (sometimes they would take the van to a cemetery for quiet and privacy), Terry was off again, up and down the hills of Northern Ontario, his band of collectors and the police trailing behind.

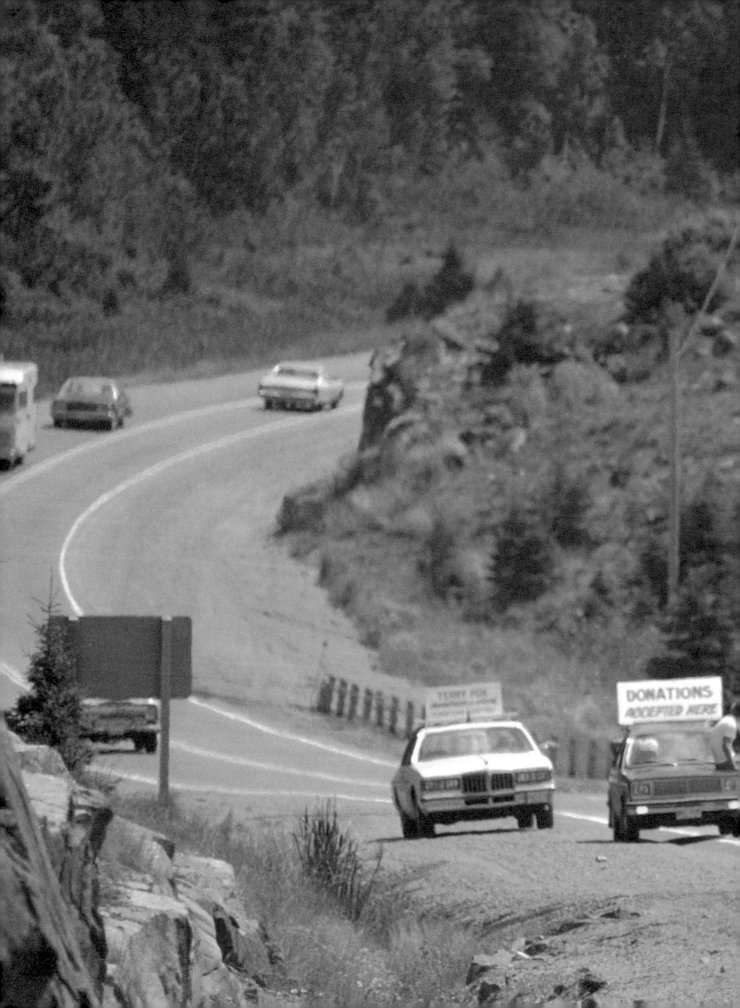

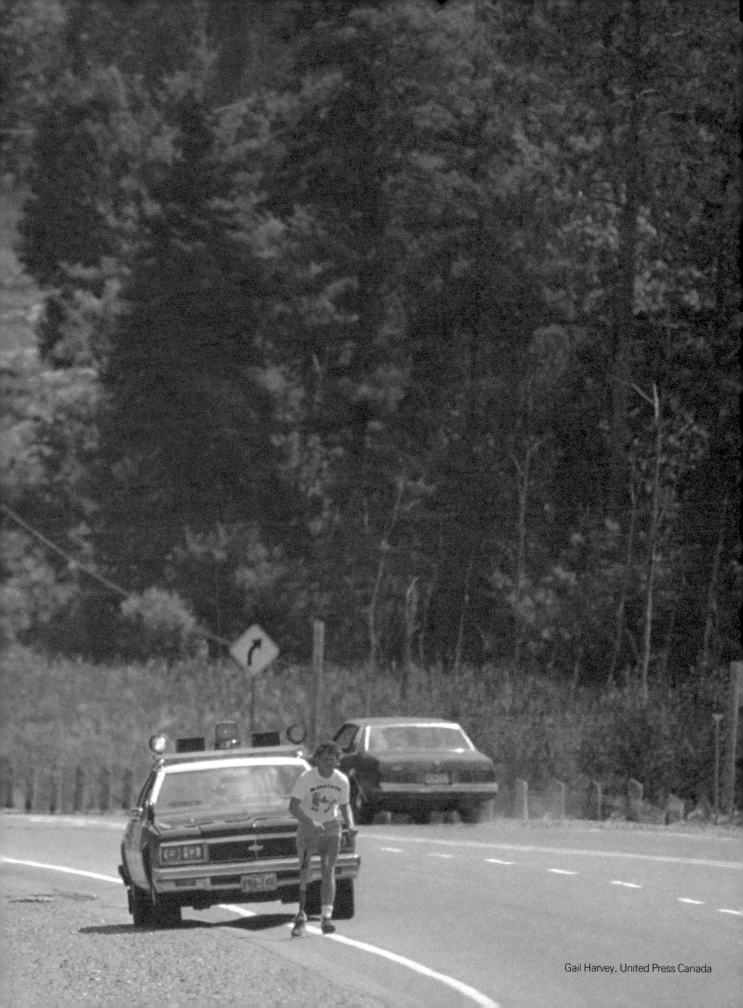

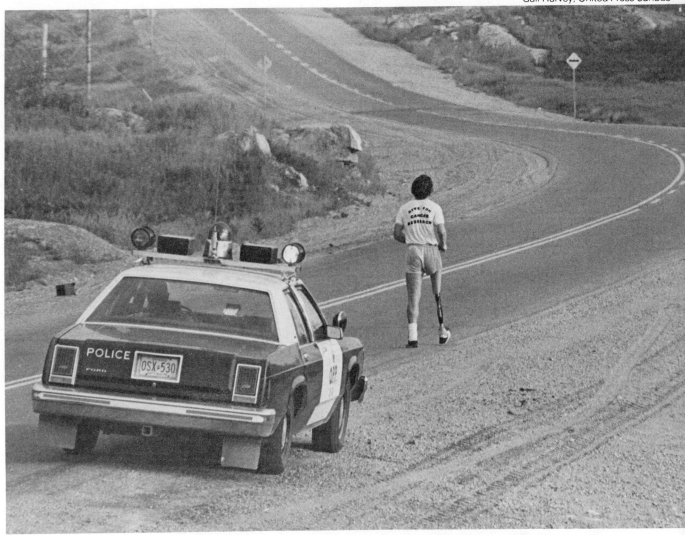

The man described as "Canada's fittest human being" had no trouble running *up* hills, just *down* hills. The reason? The artificial leg was difficult to manipulate downhill. In his pre-run training in B.C., Terry had run up various hills time and time again to build strength and endurance. He also became a member of Canada's national wheelchair basketball team, one of the top ones in the world. He and a friend would sometimes wheel their chairs two miles up a steep hill near Simon Fraser University, then drive back and do it again. (He didn't 'wheel' down; when he did that he would wreck the wheelchair tire.) As the rolling hills began to appear in the north, this writer was told Terry had no trouble completing his twenty-six miles, and that the hills proved no problem. The raw beauty of the Precambrian Shield country was outstanding.

But the inevitable lines of cars that would form behind him (right) were not simply waiting to pass, nor were they there for the magnificent scenery. They were there to watch the *wunderkind*.

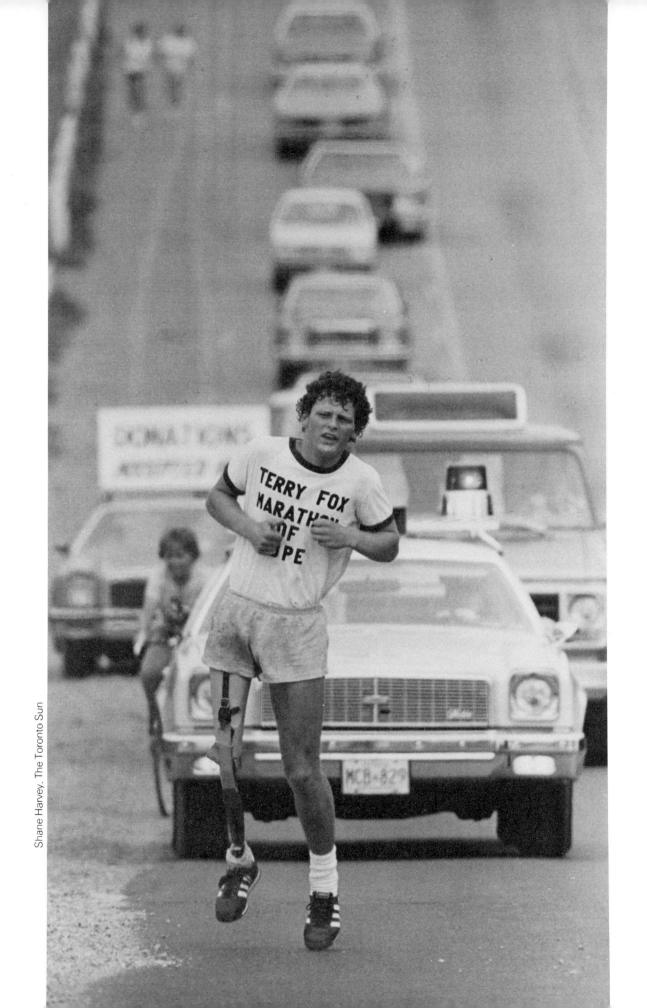

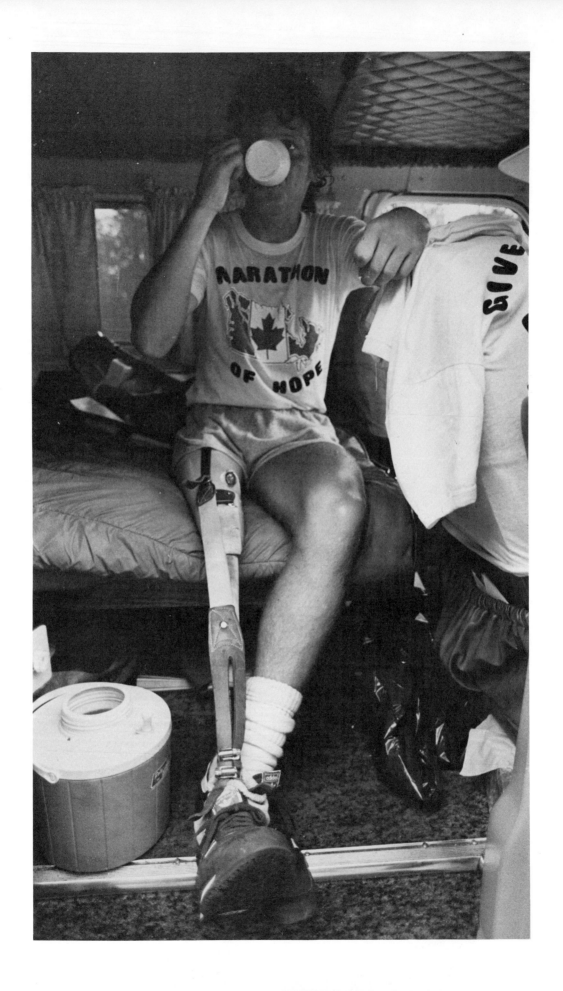

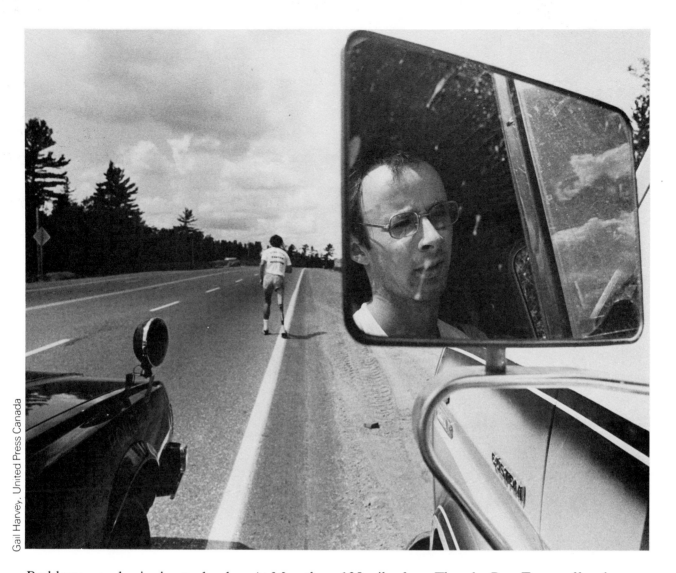

Problems were beginning to develop. At Marathon, 135 miles from Thunder Bay, Terry suffered a swollen ankle. He was rushed to Terrace Bay and the nearest airport, then flown to Sault Ste. Marie for an examination in hospital. The diagnosis was tendonitis, an inflammation of the tendons in the ankle. Two days were lost. He resumed from the place he had left off, and the run continued. At this point the total donated had passed $1,100,000. While Terry had set no specific target, he had hoped to raise a million dollars. He later revised that to a dollar for every Canadian. Near Sudbury, Terry instructed his group to take the shortest routes, by-passing, if necessary, cities and towns. At Sault Ste. Marie, a spring popped in the knee of his artificial leg. A mechanic was brought in to make repairs. Then, some ninety miles north of Sault Ste. Marie, at Montreal River Harbour on the shore of Lake Superior, Terry developed a cough. The consensus was that Terry had a cold. The hills were tough. Running toward Nipigon, the weather was very cool, and the cough didn't stop. The rain which dogged the run at this portion, continued.

But the day-to-day routine of the run appeared normal. Rest stops for water (left), back on the road with Doug at the wheel (above). Receptions were held, and donations flowed in from everywhere.

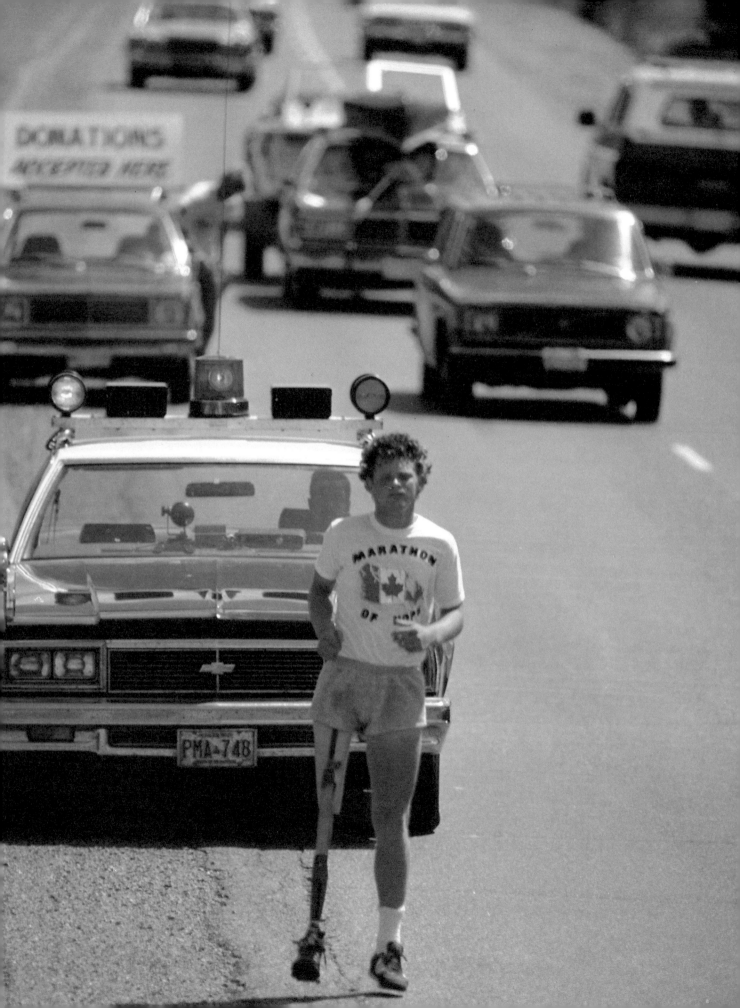

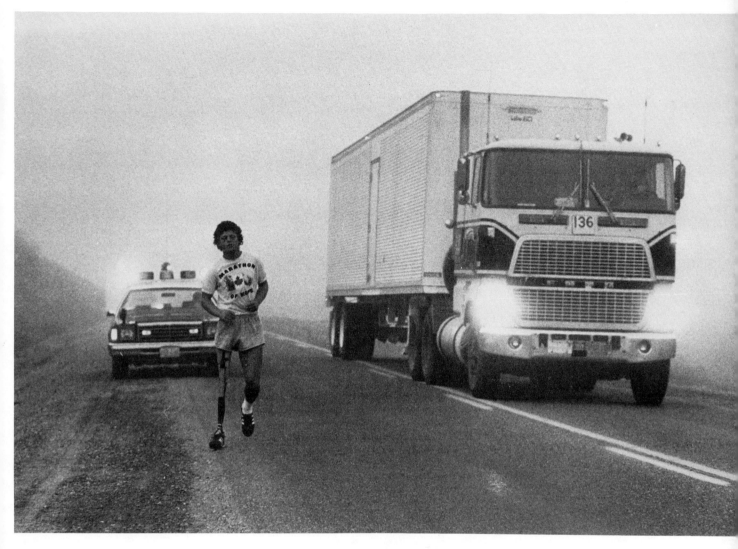

"I thought something might be wrong," said Vigars. Terry, prophetically, had said during various earlier interviews things like " . . . if I can finish the run . . . if something happens I can't control . . . "

But no one with the entourage thought for a second the "something wrong" would be anything more than a severe cold.

The run continued . . . and so did the cough.

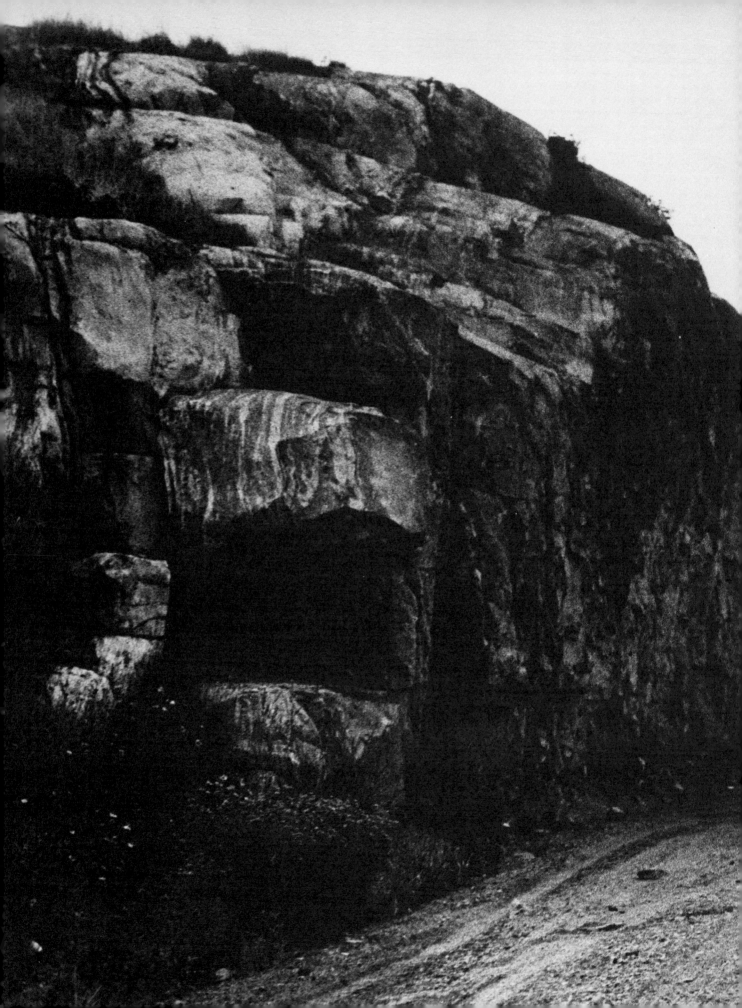

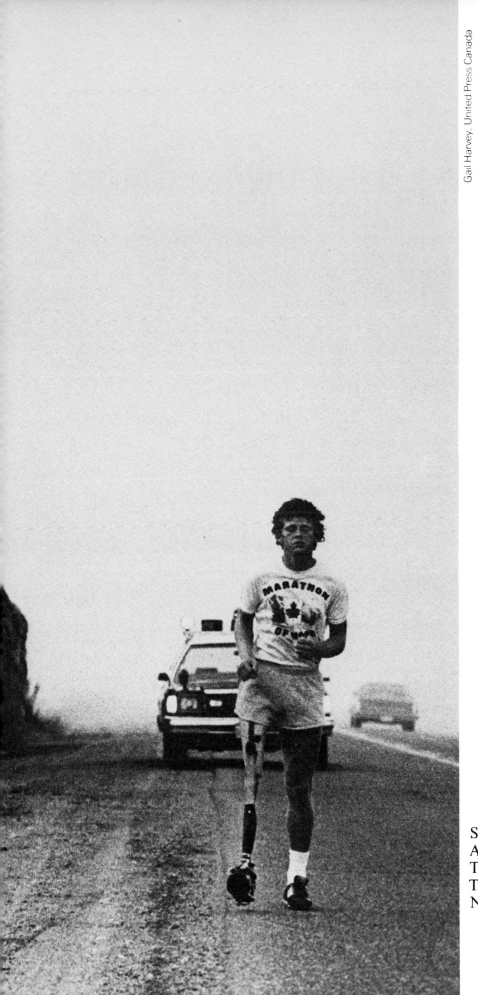

Gail Harvey, United Press Canada

Sunday, August 30.
A great day.
Terry ran twenty-six miles.
The cough vanished.
No signs of a cold.

Monday, September 1, Labour Day. Up at four a.m., on the road by five. For the first eighteen miles there were no problems, but the cough returned. Terry took a break, and went to the van. He fell asleep.

After the break, he ran another three miles, close to the Thunder Bay by-pass, then stopped and climbed into the van. It was untypical. He again fell asleep. Not long after, he was awakened. The cars of people were waiting to see him. Terry clambered out. They tried to dissuade him from running. "I owe it to them," he replied. He ran another mile, until he ran out of cars.

Then he said, "Take me to a hospital."

Darrell, Doug and Lou Fine, the district director, raced into Thunder Bay. Terry changed his mind. Not hospital, but to a hotel. Then to hospital. The doctor diagnosed a collapsed lung, and fluid was building. X-rays showed two spots, one on each lung. The conversation went something like this.

Terry: "Is it cancer?"

Doctor: "Well, I can't be sure until I do further tests."

Terry: "Tell me the truth. Is it cancer?"

It was. His world exploded.

Betty and Rolly Fox were at home in Port Coquitlam. They raced to the airport and were in Thunder Bay the morning of September 2. Bill Vigars was in Welland. He didn't sleep all night and caught the early flight to Thunder Bay. Later, Bill related to this writer the following impressions and sequence of events.

"So I didn't sleep that night at all. Air Canada was able to get me on a flight at seven, that was the Tuesday morning because it happened on Labour Day. I showed up in Thunder Bay about an hour after his mum and dad had flown in from B.C. We sat and waited, and then his mum and dad were called down, and Darrell and I wandered around. Doug was across the street. Darrell and I went down and sat outside the doctor's office, and when they came out we could tell what it was. Terry had already been taken back to his room. His mum, dad and Darrell went in first; then about two minutes later they came out and got me. That was rather a difficult time. Terry hates hospital food, so after all the tests were done and the problem confirmed as cancer, we received permission to take him out to a restaurant. I was on the telephone across the street in the Cancer Lodge. Terry walked out with his mum and dad; we were going to drive down in the camper. As I walked over he was standing there, and all of a sudden his legs went out from underneath him. His dad caught him and I came running. We grabbed him and started carrying him back to the hospital. At this point his mum got quite upset. His dad left to take care of her and I ended up carrying Terry into the hospital. He couldn't breathe and was coughing. The doctor saw us coming and got him to a stretcher. He was in something like a waiting room, a treatment room, and he was very white and couldn't seem to breathe."

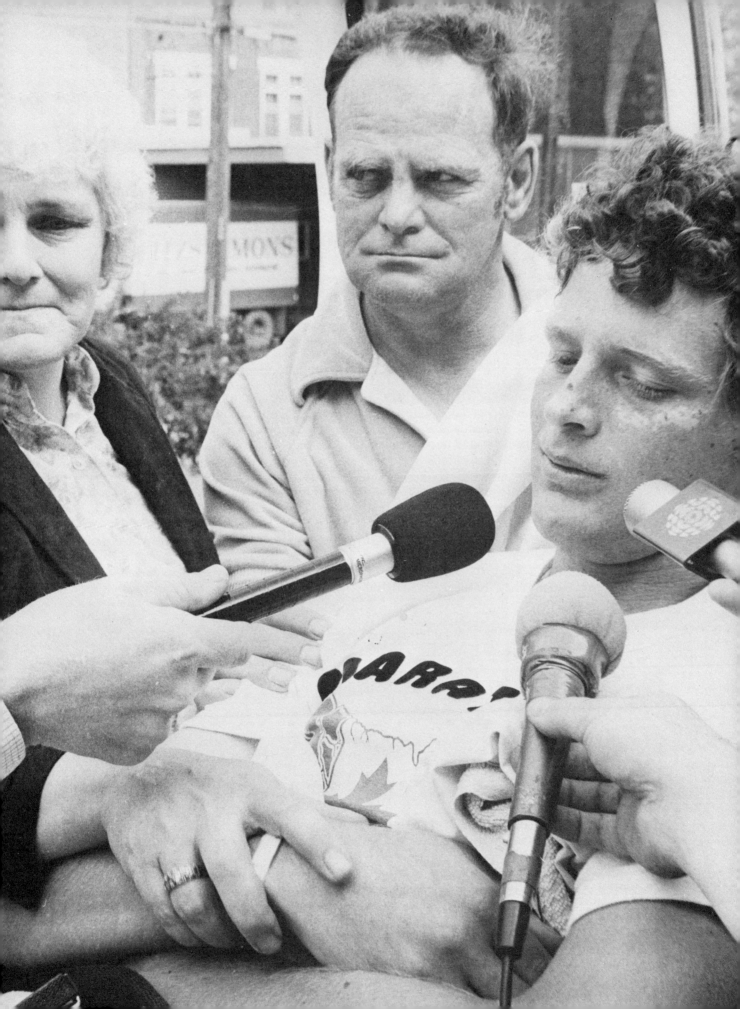

Tuesday, September 2.

The *Toronto Star* sent a Lear jet from Toronto with reporter Christie Blatchford and photographer David Cooper. Would the *Star* use that jet to take Terry home? It wasn't possible. A public health nurse and Lou Fine called the Ministry of Health. Quickly, a plan was hatched to spread the cost between OHIP and British Columbia. A second Lear jet left Toronto International Airport. They raced each other to Thunder Bay. A brief press conference was held in which Terry told the world he had cancer of the lungs and had to return home.

He said, "I didn't think this would happen, it was an unbelievable shock. I mean, I've been doing great, doing those twenty-six miles every day, up those hills, I had less than 2,000 to go. I thought I was lucky as I was going so great."

"Well, you know I had primary cancer in my knee 3½ years ago, and now the cancer is in my lungs . . . (The voice seems to crack a little) . . . and I really have to go home and have some more treatment. I have to go home and have some more X-rays and maybe an operation that will involve opening up my chest, or more drugs. I'll do everything I can. I'm gonna do my very best, I'll fight, I promise I won't give up."

The prognosis was not revealed. It was very bad. The osteogenic sarcoma had come to rest in the lungs and was metastasising. Going wild. It was a virulent cancer.

The deep agony evident in their faces, Betty and Rolly Fox sat by their son. Betty, the strong-willed compassionate mother. Rolly, the competitive, loving, concerned father, a railway switchman for the CNR. Their precious son, grieviously ill.

The ambulance screamed out to the airport. Terry was lifted gently into the Lear. Betty, Rolly and Bill Vigars embraced, tears flowing. Bill and Terry hugged for the longest time. They boarded quickly with a doctor who was there in case an emergency tracheotomy was necessary, because of the collapsed lung and the fluid buildup. As Bill watched the jet leave, the tears lingered on. Darrell and Doug took a commercial jet home. Both flights arrived within minutes of each other. Fred met them at the airport. Terry's plane parked in the distance, away from press and gawkers. He was rushed to Royal Columbian Hospital where Dr. Ladislav Antonik, on the case from the very beginning, patiently waited.

Bill Vigars caught the 11.00 p.m. National News. He was dumbfounded. There were Terry, Betty and Rolly (right) giving a press conference earlier the same evening at the hospital, after the exhausting 2,000 mile flight. It was an unbelievable day.

Terry's marathon was over. His Marathon of Hope will never end.

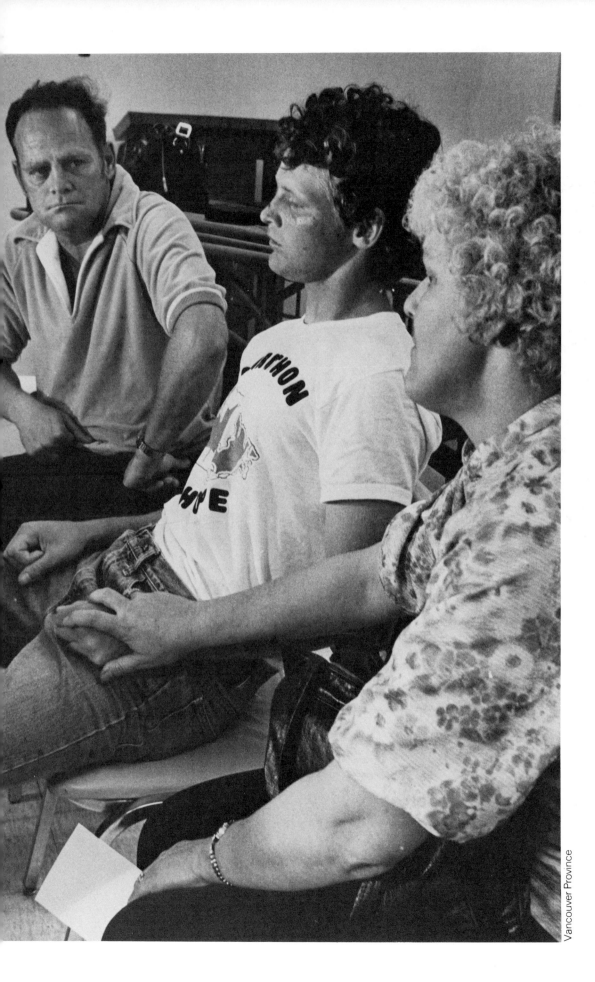

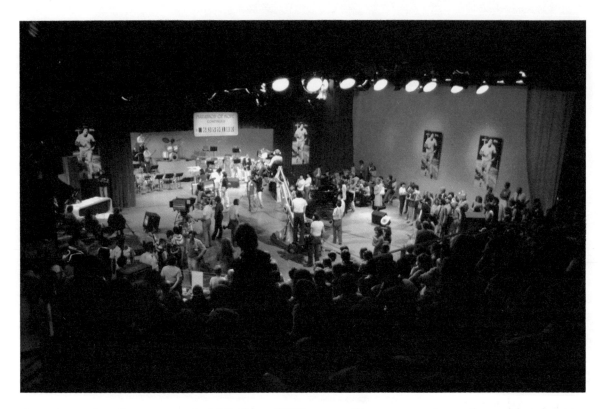

As a stunned nation mourned, Al Parks, a CTV news editor proposed a nation-wide telecast, not a telethon, but a tribute to Terry Fox. President Murray Chercover agreed, quickly cleared time on sixteen stations, and in an unbelievable five days mounted what turned out to be a brilliant five-hour telecast the next Sunday in prime time.

Stars from across the continent agreed to perform. John Denver, whose song *You Say The Battle's Over* was Terry's favourite, hired a camera crew in Hollywood to film a tribute. The response was incredible.

In a quickly constructed set (above), a large audience formed the backdrop to the evening. Starting with the $1,700,000 already pledged or donated, CTV took on the nation.

In Vancouver, in fact in all of British Columbia, the outpouring was spectacular. At BCTV, the CTV affiliate, the program was extended an additional two hours. At the end of the night, $1,061,394 had been pledged or donated. Outside the studio was chaos: cars, trucks, buses, tractor-trailers, motorcycles — people arrived to drop bills, cheques, jars of coins into plastic bins. Mayor Jack Volrich, actor Leslie Nielsen and Nancy Greene Raine plus scores of other celebrities attended. One young boy wanted to donate his parents' house. But he didn't know the address. Betty and Rolly Fox, with daughter Judith and brother Fred, helped man the phones. Said Rolly, "It's unbelievable." And it was.

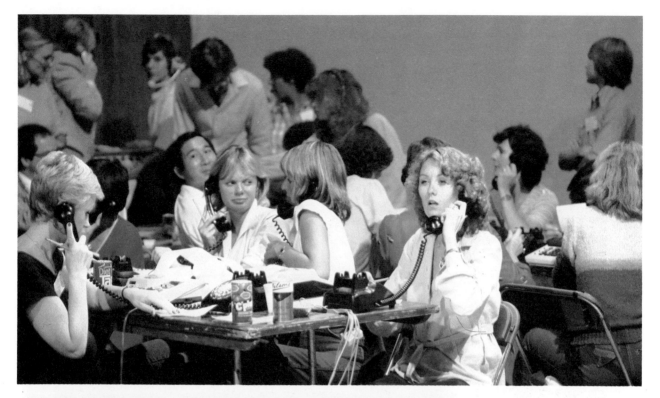

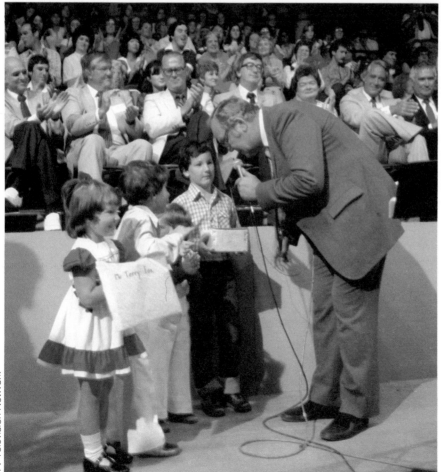

Scores of volunteers were there to take pledges at the studio (above). Elsewhere across the nation, emergency switchboards were arranged to handle calls. Bell Telephone crews worked around the clock to make the connections. It was the fastest setup anyone can recall.

Co-host Harvey Kirck (left) accepts donations from a group of children. The biggest check from a corporation was $100,000. The total rose by the minute.

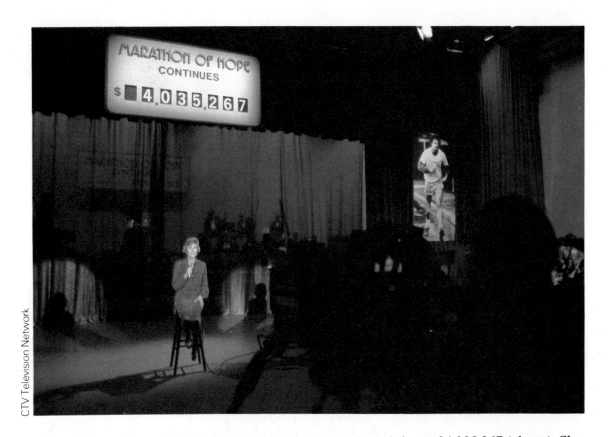

CTV Television Network

Anne Murray, in spotlight, sings for Terry as the tote board shows $4,035,267 (above). She and Glen Campbell, in Toronto for a performance, talk of the marathon. Elton John, Al Waxman, Kris Kristopherson, Nana Mouskouri, Darryl Sittler, Bobby Orr (via telephone), Betty Kennedy, Barbara Frum, Joyce Davidson, Paul Williams, an orchestra, dancers and singers from Stratford, corporate leaders—all come. One million dollars is pledged by Ontario. Another million is pledged by the province of British Columbia. By the time ballet superstars Karen Kain and Frank Augustyn appear (right) to perform an eight minute segment from Romeo and Juliet, the total is $7,374,575.

During, or after the CTV tribute, many of the affiliate stations cut in with local appeals for money. At Winnipeg's CKY, anchormen Ray Torgurd and Peter Young raised $225,000. The total in Winnipeg exceeded $600,000. Quarterbacks for the Calgary Stampeders and Winnipeg Blue Bombers showed up, Terry's uncle appeared (Terry was born in Winnipeg), and a week after the tribute the phones were still ringing at the rate of 30 calls per day.

Johnny Sandison of CKCK Regina was host, and the program there raised $250,000 in Southern Saskatchewan. The entire province: $782,000 to date, just short of $1 per person. Volunteers came from the RCMP, Cancer Society and service clubs.

At CFQC in Saskatchewan, they had a drive-in collection point outside the station. Mayor Cliff Wright and other officials collected money in baskets. Total: $235,000.

At CFCN Calgary, host Ron Barge displayed a map from Thunder Bay to Calgary showing donations per mile as they came in. The station set a target of $500,000, and when they signed off they had raised $671,000. It later increased to $762,000. Some 300 phone lines had to be installed, calling for major renovations.

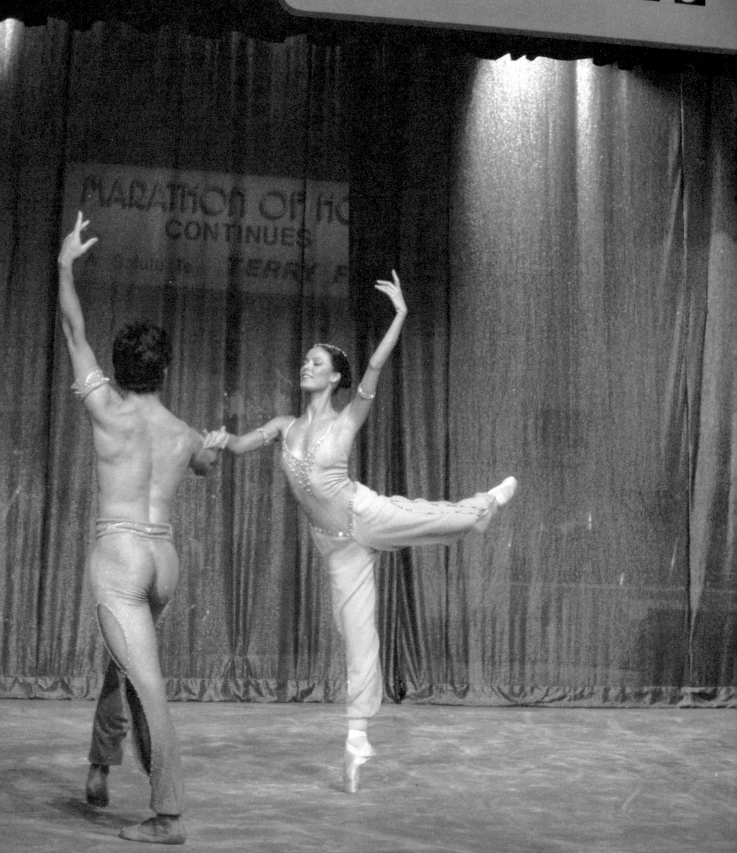

CONTINUES

$ 7,374,575

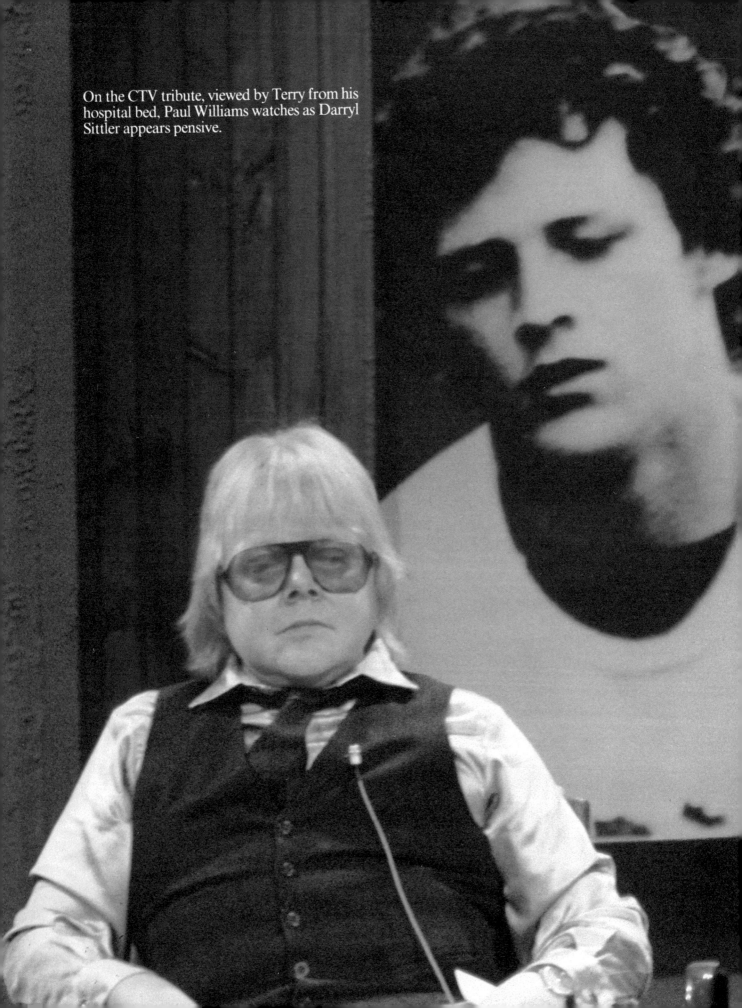

On the CTV tribute, viewed by Terry from his hospital bed, Paul Williams watches as Darryl Sittler appears pensive.

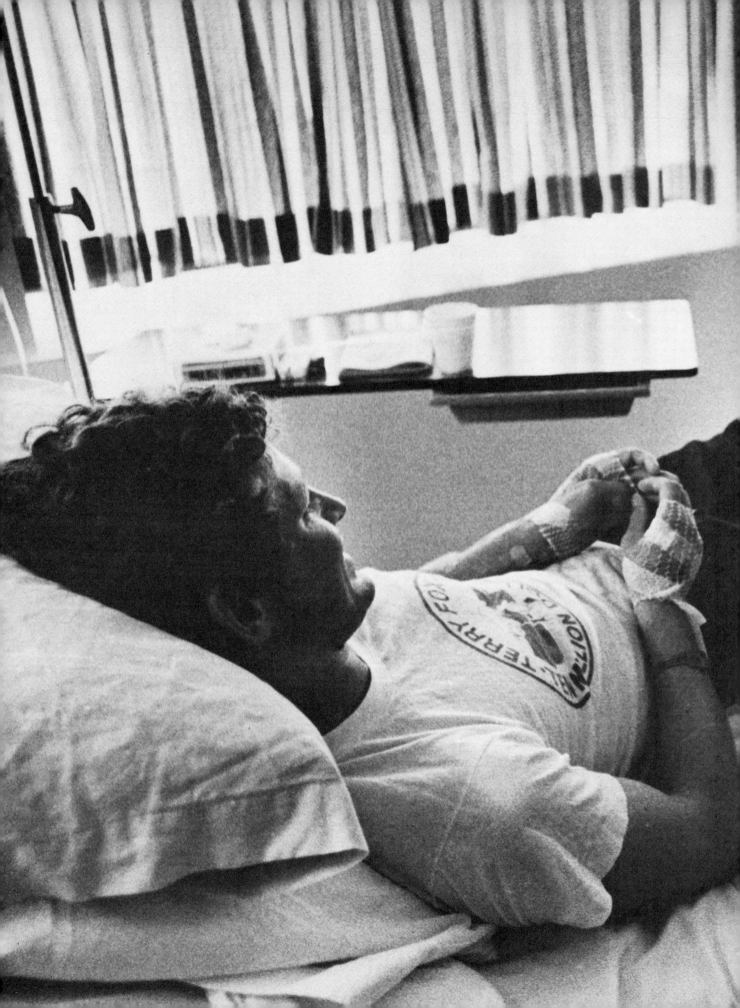

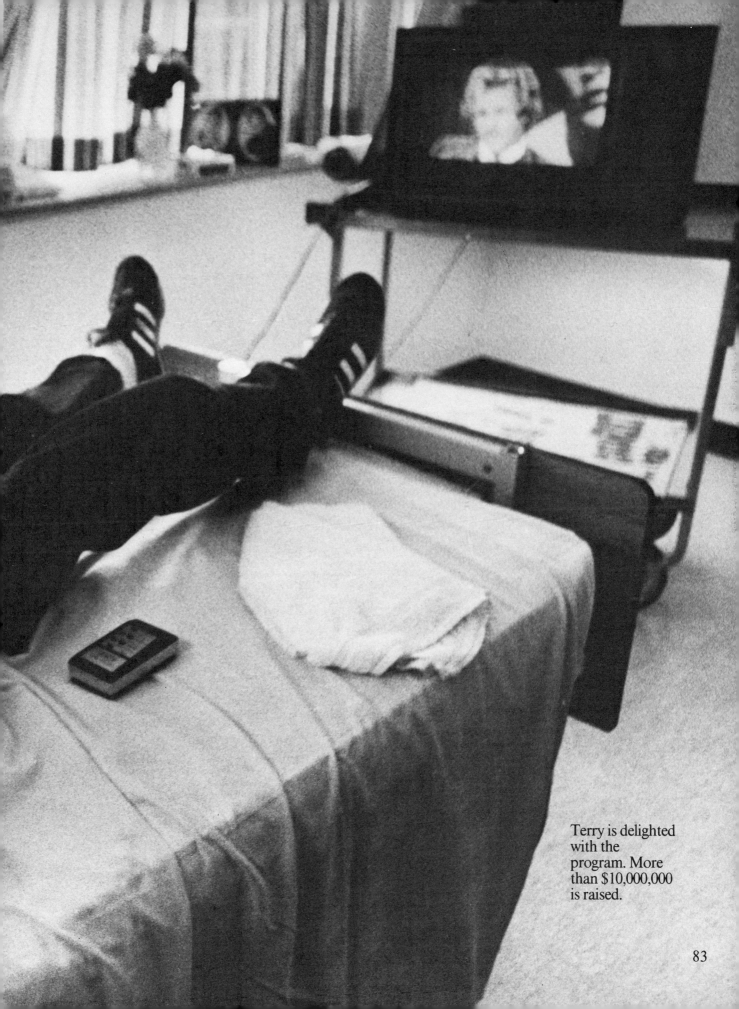

Terry is delighted
with the
program. More
than $10,000,000
is raised.

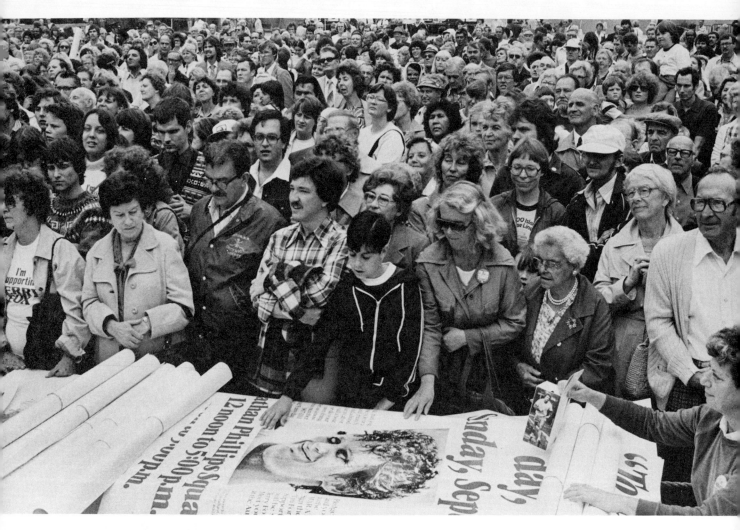

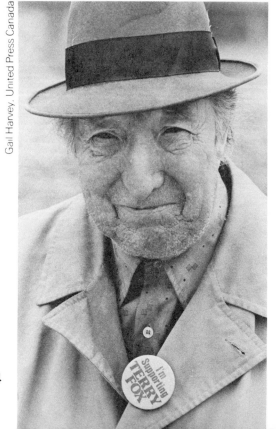

Gail Harvey. United Press Canada

The outpouring of emotion knew no bounds. People who had pledged $10 gave $100. Pledges were doubled, tripled, quadrupled. At CKFM the total was $92,000 before September 2. In the following two days $100,000 came in. But a lot of people were saying, "I've given all I can. But I want to do something more." Businessman Quentin Wahl was one. Quickly an idea jelled. We pulled together a cadre of people—the *Toronto Star,* CFTO-TV, CKFM, Southam-Murray Printing. Scores of other people and companies pitched in. Bob Little, an events organizer, proposed the title: To Terry, With Love. It was to be a participation day. The 48th Highlanders led a parade down University Avenue. There was a three-mile run. Scores of celebrities spoke to the 15,000 people who turned up over the four-hour event. A 'support-o-gram' was signed by thousands of people and sent to Terry. His recorded voice was played to the crowds.

"I will always remember Toronto as . . . the area of Canada where the Marathon of Hope really took off. I remember the people here as being fantastic . . . and from here on, in every town and city I went to, we had a tremendous response. . .

"So, I'd really like to thank all of you people who have come out and hope that you will continue doing the fund raising and having the spirit that you have now."

People brought posters, drawings of Terry, and donated money. It was a Sunday, September 21, and the Canadian Imperial Bank of Commerce opened a nearby branch to take in money donated. More than $40,000 was received there, and perhaps another $20,000 from the sale of buttons around Toronto, organized by Jack Creed. Donald Sutherland, the famous actor, gave the last speech, a moving and compelling tribute. It was quite a day.

Vancouver, in the radio field, went wild. The first station to offer support was CJOR, which ran weekly reports from Terry on the road. As the momentum grew, CJOR raised more than $80,000. CKNW, before the recurrence of cancer, had organized a Terry Fox night at a B.C. Lions football game. The tribute continued. Terry was able to attend. CFMI-FM received a spontaneous outburst from its listeners, who gave more than $30,000. All radio and TV stations supported the effort. Terry, of course, was British Columbia's native son.

In Toronto, radio station Q-107 earlier held a twenty-four hour telethon in which announcer Scruff Connors raised $150,000.

Right across the nation, school children, service clubs, small and large industries indulged in a mind-boggling array of activities to raise money: runs, walks, crawls, parties, car washings, lake cruises. People supplied goods, services and cash. It was beyond anyone's wildest expectations.

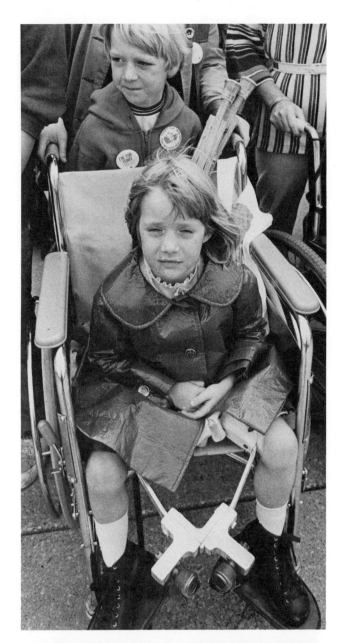

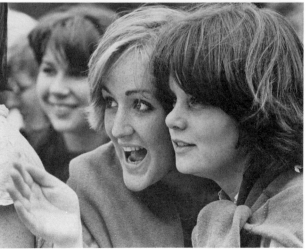

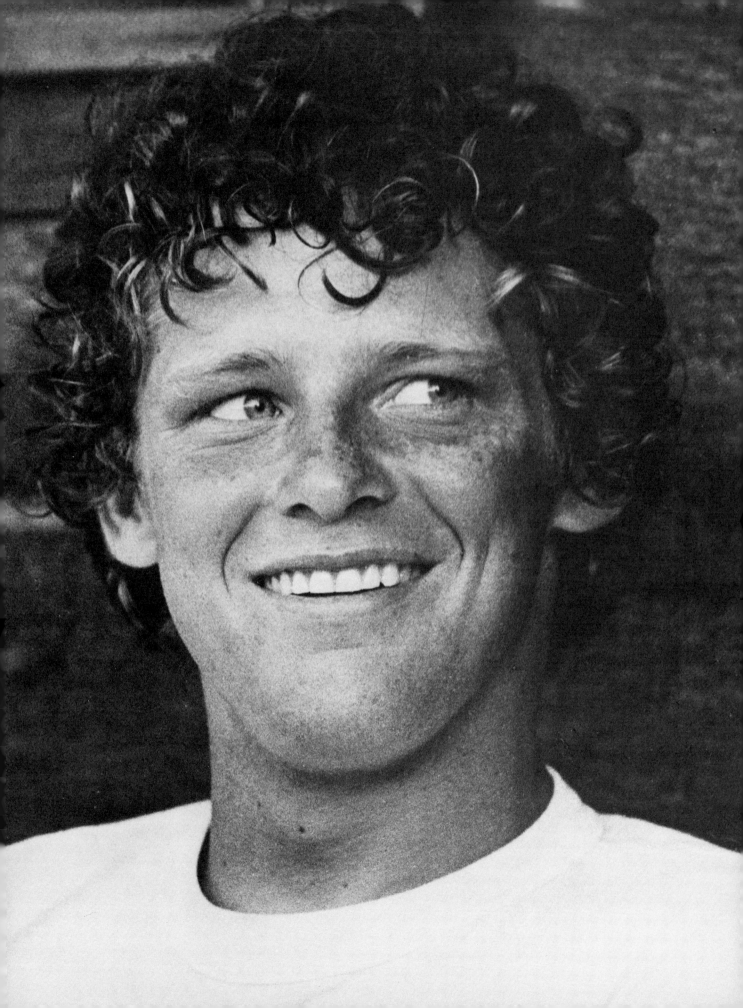

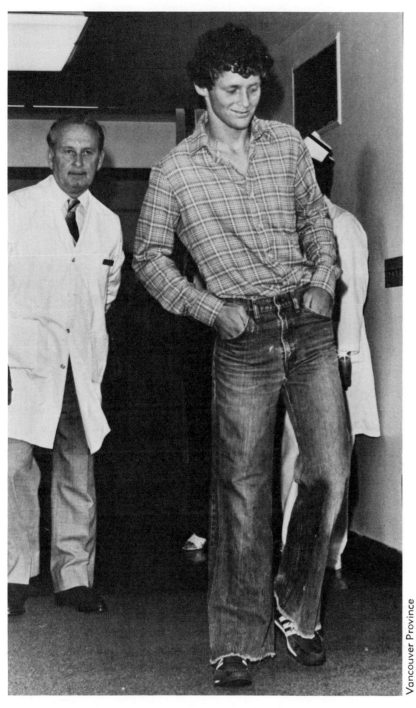

Vancouver Province

September 5. Chemotherapy began, this time with the drugs Leukovorin,
Cis-platinum, Vincristine and Methotrexate. The treatment was painful. After the
initial effects passed, he was released to go home to Port Coquitlam and convalesce. Above, Terry
leaves the hospital with Dr. Ladislav Antonik and Head Nurse Allison Sinson. The drugs were
administered to stop the spread of cancer, hopefully shrink it, and provide a chance to operate on the
tumours. Every three to four weeks, he would be re-examined, tested, and given another dose of
chemotherapy. In between, it was private drives, a visit to a pub, and rest. The mail, letters, telegrams,
poems and gifts filled the house. The family closed around him tightly.

Following thousands of requests, a hastily-convened Advisory Council to the Order of Canada voted Terry a Companion of the Order, Canada's highest award. Governor General Ed Schreyer made the presentation in Port Coquitlam's tiny City Hall, as the event was carried live on Canadian and U.S. television.

Below, Schreyer bestows the medal.

Right, Terry sits with his mother.

Later, Terry was given the Order of the Dogwood, British Columbia's highest honour, by Premier Bill Bennett.

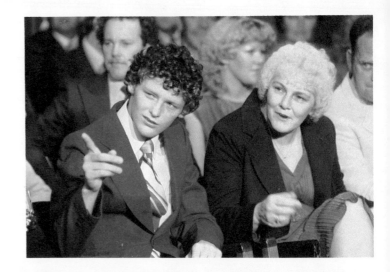

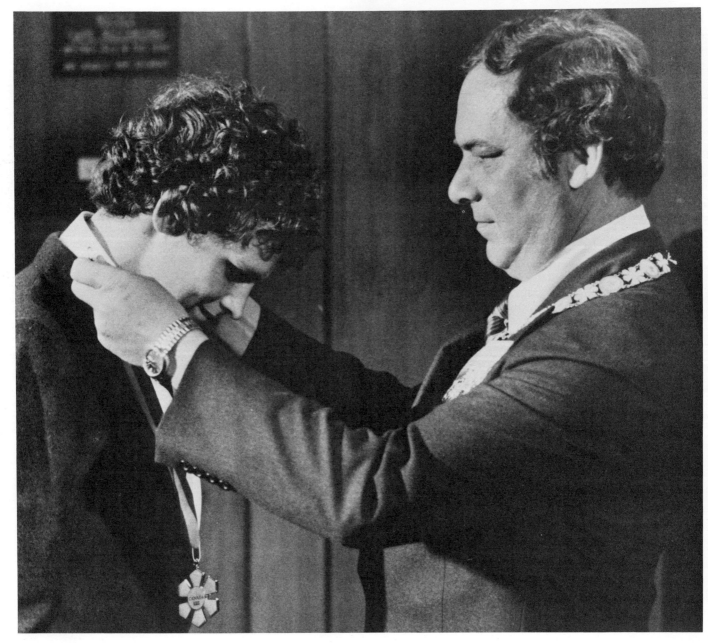

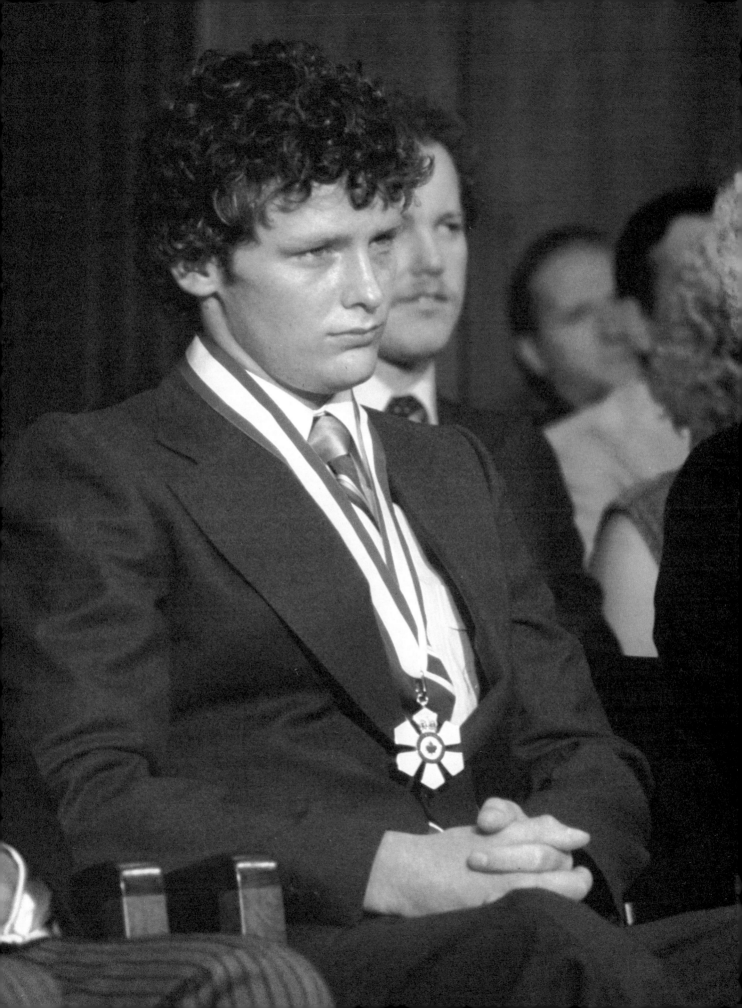

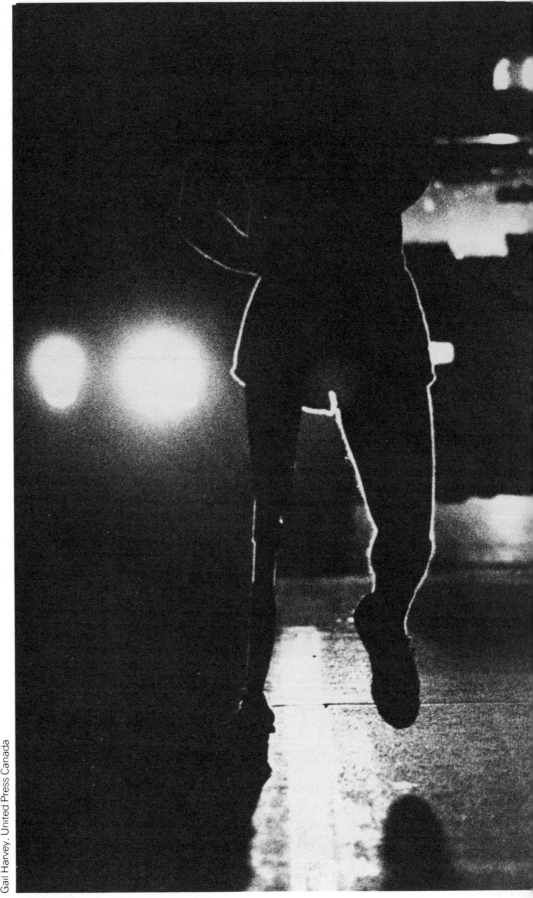

Gail Harvey. United Press Canada

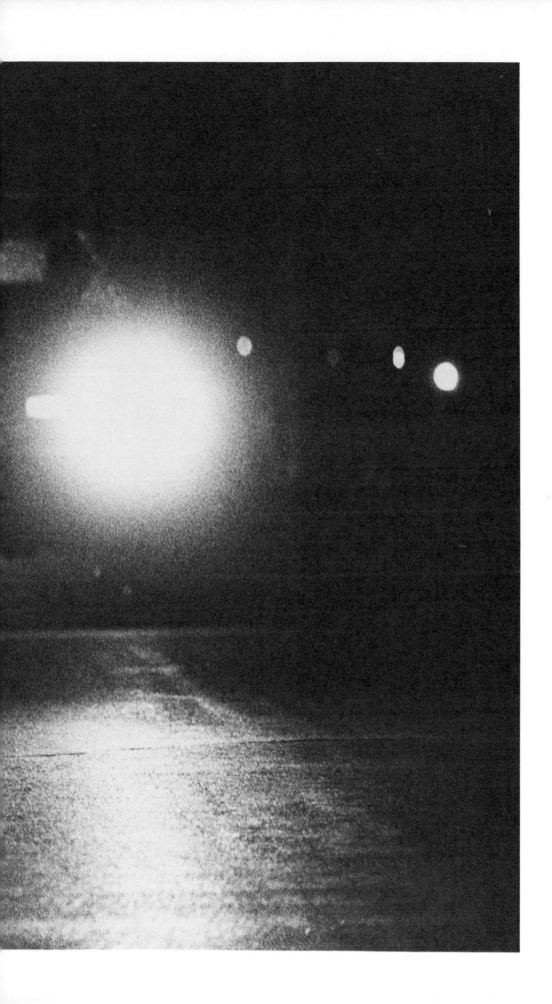

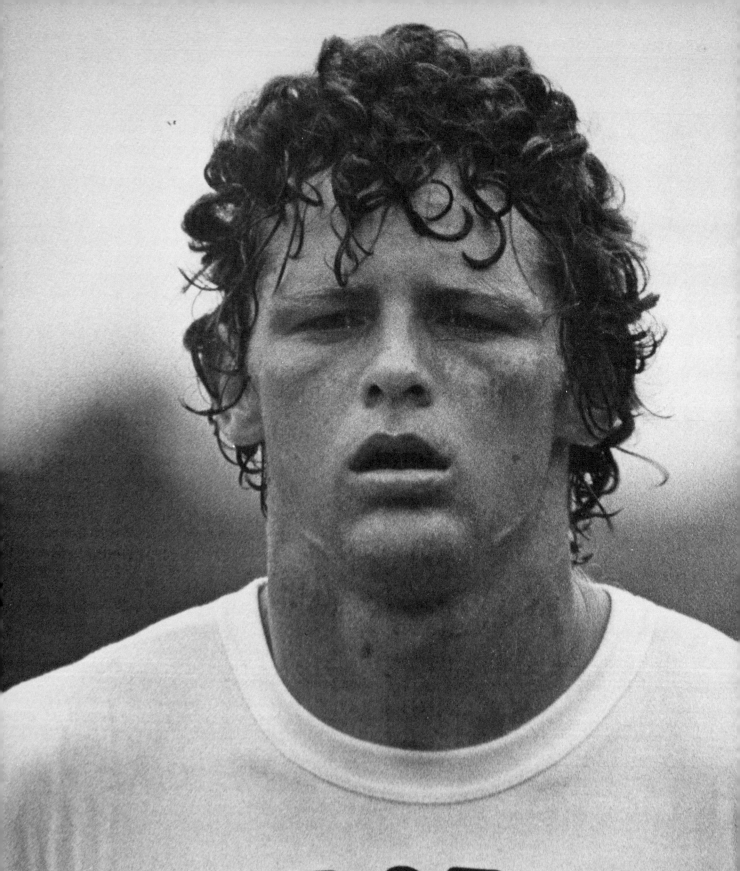

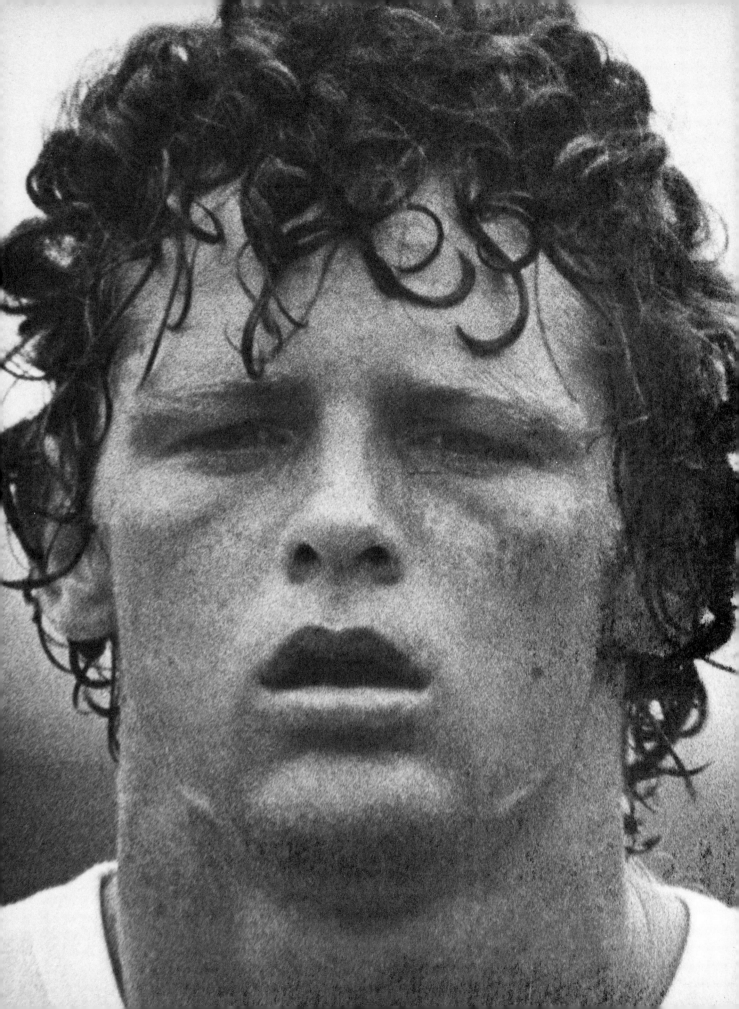

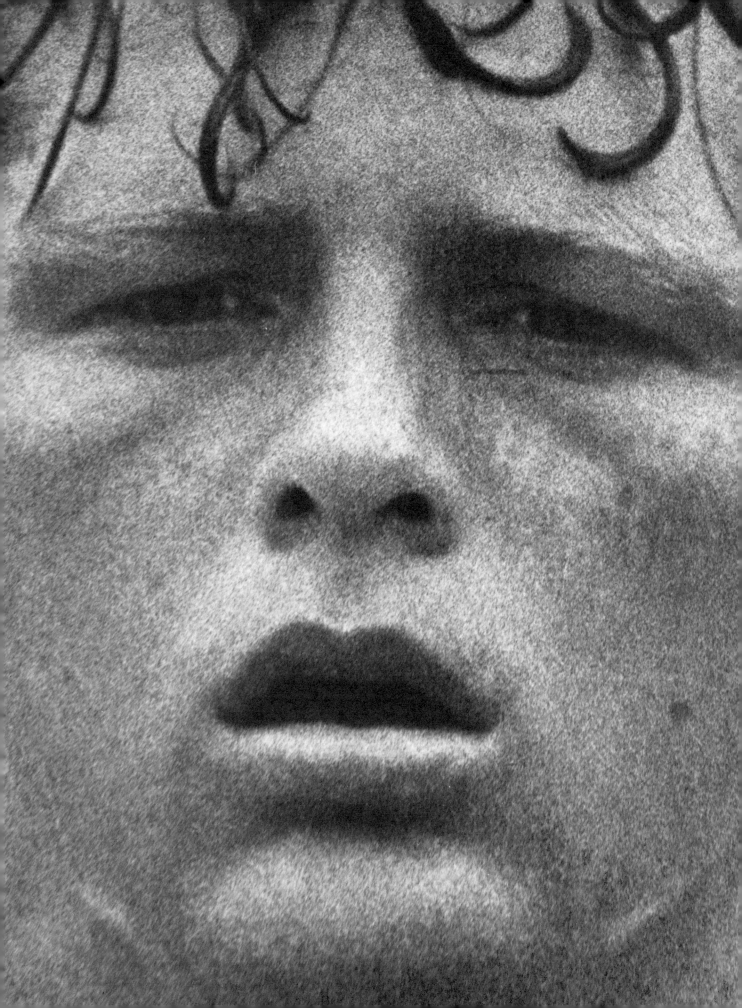